UNDERGROUND CURES

The Most Urgent Health Discoveries of 1998

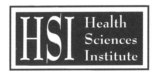

HSI Health Sciences Institute

Agora Health Books

Publisher: Kathleen Peddicord

Managing Editor: Shannon Finch

Copy Editor: Ken Danz

Table of Contents

Introduction

*E*very day, around the world, researchers and scientists are making exciting medical breakthroughs and health discoveries. Yet, you are often deprived of these healing possibilities. Your doctor may be too busy to sift through all the latest research. Or maybe he is overly influenced by the big pharmaceutical companies. Or perhaps a potentially lifesaving treatment is trapped in the tangles of government bureaucracy. The bottom line is this — for one reason or another, you are not getting the health information you need when you need it.

Underground Cures *brings together the most urgent health discoveries of the year from the world's most progressive health clinics and research laboratories. Within these pages, you will find a hidden universe of remedies and healing possibilities you never imagined existed. The mainstream medical establishment and even many alternative medical communities have yet to discover these advanced, underground cures and urgent health breakthroughs.*

Underground Cures *is packed with secrets for enhancing your health, extending your life, and liberating yourself from the devastating effects of many serious conditions. In Section I, you will learn how to achieve super immunity using natural immune-system boosters. Section II discusses the power of panaceas — natural remedies that can restore your health and vitality and offer you relief from a wide range of conditions. Section III reveals breakthrough solutions and underground cures for chronic conditions, including depression, arthritis, and herpes. Finally, in Section IV, you will be introduced to several health-enhancing, cutting-edge technologies.*

In 1996, nearly a dozen conventionally and holistically trained doctors formed a network through which they could rapidly exchange news of the latest, most innovative cures and overcome bureaucratic blocks and delays. This network is the Health Sciences Institute, dedicated to uncovering and researching the most urgent advances in modern underground medicine, like those in this book. The hard work and commitment of these "underground" health pioneers brings these cures to light . . . so that you can use them today.

The Health Sciences Institute now has over 60,000 members worldwide. As it grows in international reputation, more and more laboratories and scientists send news of their research directly to the Institute. The editors at HSI research the truly revolutionary breakthroughs for safety, efficacy, and availability.

Every day, stacks of letters arrive from people whose lives were turned around by something uncovered by HSI. The Institute maintains a file of members who have overcome diseases such as arthritis, prostate disorders, fatigue, and depression — of members who, although they had given up hope, decided to give it one last shot using a remedy they read about in an HSI publication. Please turn to page 179 to find out how you can receive regular news of the latest medical breakthroughs by becoming a member of the Health Sciences Institute.

Section I

Four Secrets to Achieving Super Immunity

*I*n today's world, we are constantly assaulted by a growing number of environmental and biological threats to our health. There's simply no way to avoid the drug-resistant bacteria, industrial chemicals, and nutrient-depleted foods that depress our natural immune responses and leave us vulnerable. The best defense? To develop disease resistance at the cellular level — in short, to achieve super immunity.

In this chapter, you'll learn about a new generation of natural immune-system boosters that may provide the most effective health insurance you can buy. Read on to learn how you can resist and overcome the most serious health threats of our age.

Chapter I

The Lactoferrin Miracle

Lactoferrin is one of the rare healing substances that inspire us — and permit us — to take a good look into the bright future of medicine. The wonderful news is that we're on the verge of a major medical breakthrough.

Because of this unique extract, much of what we now consider state-of-the-art medicine — such as radiation, antibiotics, and chemotherapy — may eventually seem as primitive and absurd as bloodletting.

If lactoferrin proves to be as powerful as its promise, many deadly diseases that haunt our thoughts today will no longer frighten us. Even fast-spreading cancers — which most doctors are helpless to restrain — could soon become as innocuous and manageable as a 24-hour bug.

Where does lactoferrin come from and how does it work?

From the moment you were born, lactoferrin — an iron-binding protein found in mother's first milk (colostrum) — was your first shield against infection and disease and your primary source of immune-system chemicals.

The primary task of your immune system is to survey your body — organ by organ, tissue by tissue, cell by cell — and make sure that only the cells that are supposed to be there. . . are there. When a strong, healthy immune system recognizes a foreign substance — a virus or cancerous cell, for example — it immediately goes into action to eliminate it.

Researchers discovered the significance of lactoferrin to the immune system while researching a mysterious biological phenomenon: pregnancy.

What's so mysterious about pregnancy?

Until recently, scientists had been baffled by the fact that a woman's body doesn't normally reject a fetus, which naturally contains the foreign antigens of the father. But the puzzle is beginning to unravel: Science has discovered that shortly after conception, a woman's immune system is down-regulated. This is why her body does not reject the fetus as "foreign" matter. (For this reason, pregnant women should not take lactoferrin.) Immediately after delivery, however, her body produces colostrum, or first milk, which restores her immune system. . . and provides powerful immune chemicals to the infant. Lactoferrin is the primary immune-system chemical in first milk.

Studies have shown that a mother's first milk is literally the only way for an infant to get these significant immune substances. Synthetic formulas cannot offer the same nutritional, immunological, or physiological value, despite efforts to produce formulas that mimic breast milk as closely as possible.

How critical are these immune factors?

Research has shown that in both developed and undeveloped countries, infants who are not breast-fed suffer higher rates of childhood infections and tend to have higher incidences of iron-deficiency anemia. Studies also show that people with lactoferrin deficiencies succumb early in their lives to infections that most people routinely fight off.

But lactoferrin provides a unique benefit for people of all ages. As an adult, your body continues to produce this immune chemical. It's found in secretions like tears, perspiration, the lining of the intestinal tract, and the mucous membranes that line the nose, ears, throat, and urinary tract — all the places that are especially vulnerable to infection.

It's also found in certain white blood cells, called neutrophils, that surround and kill bacteria and viruses. We know, for example, that a systemic bacterial infection is accompanied by a rapid rise in lactoferrin. Whenever your skin is cut, for example, white blood cells are drawn to the area, where they release granules containing lactoferrin. The lactoferrin binds iron, which immediately halts the bacterial growth.

Lactoferrin also acts as an antioxidant — and, like any antioxidant, it works to prevent free radicals from destroying cells in your body.

Unraveling the healing mystery of lactoferrin

Lactoferrin has at least two specific functions that boost your immune system:

(1) It binds iron in your blood, keeping it away
      from cancer cells, bacteria, viruses, and
      other pathogens that require iron to grow.
      (All cells need iron to grow.)

The lactoferrin protein is able to sequester and release iron as needed, under controlled conditions. This
property helps prevent harmful oxidative reactions,
making lactoferrin a powerful antioxidant.

(2) It switches on the genes that launch your
      body's immune response.

Research suggests that the lactoferrin protein,
through a fascinating process called transcriptional
activation, activates very specific strands of DNA that
turn on the genes that launch your immune response.
This is such a rare and surprising action that there is
no category of protein like it. Lactoferrin is literally in
a class by itself!

Lactoferrin also contains antibodies against a wide
range of bacterial, fungal, viral, and protozoal pathogens. In effect, the lactoferrin protein backs budding
cancer cells or bacteria into a corner. . . starves them. . .
and sends out a signal to your white blood cells that
says, "It's over here! Come get it!"

State-of-the-art techniques in cellular and molecular biology have recently allowed us to isolate
lactoferrin from the "first food of life." The commer-
cially available preparation is in a form in which the
food has not been chemically altered.

So far, it's had astonishing results.

Lactoferrin and cancer

Researchers at New York University and Harvard University have conducted extensive research into the actions and benefits of lactoferrin. They found that lactoferrin works even better than synthetic compounds that bind free iron (a treatment used for leukemia). They also found that lactoferrin works against solid tumors. But, most importantly, it appears to work against metastasis, the deadliest phase of cancer and often the hardest to treat.

One of the Health Sciences Institute's own panel members uses lactoferrin as a crucial part of a total immune-boosting regimen for cancer patients — with astonishing results. One woman suffering from an aggressive lung cancer had been told that her case was hopeless. When she began taking lactoferrin, she was already down to 85 pounds. She was extremely weak, felt nauseated, and was breathing with difficulty.

Within weeks of starting treatment, she began to regain her strength and started to gain weight. Today, more than a year after she was told she had only a short period of time to live, she is still alive and going strong. Her seemingly miraculous recovery is due in large part to the healing power of lactoferrin.

Lactoferrin in stroke recovery

A member of the HSI network had suffered three strokes by the age of 68. After two days of lactoferrin supplementation, she reports, "I was in the house cooking, doing everything I'd always done. I'm still taking my medication for my heart attack, but I feel great! I have a lot of energy.

"Before, I couldn't speak plainly because of the stroke, but I can talk now! My speech... has come back. Also, I hadn't been able to drive because my eyesight has been so bad, but after a short time on the lactoferrin, I can drive again!"

Lactoferrin appears to have a profound effect on degenerative (as opposed to infectious) disease. Although we can't say yet exactly how, it's very possible that lactoferrin's antioxidant action plays a key role. As you know, free radicals oxidize the LDL (bad) cholesterol, which causes arteries to harden and circulation to suffer.

Lactoferrin and AIDS

After 15 years and more than $22 billion spent on research, the medical community is still struggling to develop viable treatments for AIDS. In one study of AIDS patients with chronic diarrhea (one of the first signs of the deterioration of health), the use of lactoferrin resulted in complete remission of diarrhea in 40 percent of the participants, with 24 percent experiencing partial remission (*Clinical Investigator*, no. 70, 1992, pp. 558).

We can begin to understand lactoferrin's healing abilities when we consider that, during early stages, the HIV-infected immune system displays elevated levels of a substance called isoferritin. Isoferritin is present in the maternal serum and uterine environment during pregnancy (the time when the mother's immune system is temporarily "down-regulated"). When the pregnancy is over, lactoferrin suppresses the isoferritin and the immune system returns to normal. People suffering from certain lymphomas, leukemia, breast cancer, renal disease, or celiac disease also have elevated levels of isoferritin. This means that lactoferrin may play a pivotal role in the treatment of these diseases.

Hope for autistic and brain-damaged children

Lactoferrin may even hold significant hope for children with autism or brain injuries. Nutritional biochemist Patricia Kane of Millville, New Jersey, has begun working with autistic and brain-injured children and has witnessed surprising results with the administration of lactoferrin. Although autism is a brain dysfunction, Dr. Kane points out that, because of the involvement of the entire body, improvement can only come about by embracing all the systemic interactions — a holistic approach. The use of lactoferrin represents significant progress toward this goal.

Protection against the cryptosporidium parasites

Cryptosporidium parasites cause acute diarrhea in people with strong, healthy immune systems but can be life-threatening in those who are immune compromised. Studies published in *Infection & Immunity* (no. 61, 1993, pp. 4079) have shown that colostrum is able to ameliorate or completely eliminate the clinical symptoms of those suffering from cryptosporidiosis.

What else can you use it for?

Other studies have shown that lactoferrin. . .

- contains an **anti-inflammatory** molecule — which means it can help if you suffer from **arthritis**
- functions as an inhibitor of mammary cell growth — which means it may hold promise for prevention or treatment of **breast cancer**
- plays a role in lessening ocular disturbances — which means it may help with **vision problems**
- acts as a potent antimicrobial agent against **Candida albicans**
- shows potent antiviral activity useful in reducing your susceptibility to **herpes**

If you're wondering how safe lactoferrin is, keep in mind that it is nontoxic and is well-tolerated by nursing infants.

Should you take it as a daily preventive?

Many everyday threats wear down the immune system — from environmental toxins and emotional and physical stressors to genetic problems. Taking lactoferrin on a daily basis helps upgrade your immune system, so you can take full advantage of your natural defenses in a world full of potential health threats.

Why haven't you heard of it before?

Simple. It can't be patented. By law, no natural substance can be patented as is — and lactoferrin is already at its most powerful. . . as is.

So if a major drug company were to spend hundreds of millions of dollars to have lactoferrin approved by the FDA as a cancer treatment. . . how would it get its millions back. . . when any company can produce it? So lactoferrin is destined to remain an underground alternative to other, less natural pharmaceuticals. But it is available from a limited number of suppliers in the United States and should not be overlooked as a powerful tool in the fight against serious disease.

The wonderful truth is that your body can fend for itself. . . when given the chance. The lactoferrin treatment can give it that chance, while adding a powerful healing kick to your immune system at the same time.

Actions:
- Supplies natural antibodies
- Blocks cancer-cell nourishment
- Inhibits free-radical production
- Activates DNA that launches immune responses

Benefits:
- Acts as an immune stimulant
- Has anti-inflammatory properties
- Performs an antifungal function
- Has antiparasitic properties

A recommended amount for prevention is 100 milligrams a day taken orally at bedtime. For therapy, more than 100 milligrams a day can be used without

More Advances in Cancer Therapy

One alternative medical pioneer in California has developed a program that has actually been shown to change cancer cells back to normal, healthy cells! The Lifestar Cancer Restoration Protocol consists of a daily regimen of nontoxic nutrients and herbs, along with detoxifying and immune-boosting lifestyle changes. In one recent test case, lung cancer totally disappeared in three weeks, with no evidence of scar tissue remaining!

Most of the components of this protocol can be found in your local health food store. The core program includes the following:

- 2 teaspoons of grape-seed oil, 3 times a day
- 700 milligrams of L-methioninecapsules
- 20,000 IU natural betacarotene capsules (You can use chlorella or other green concentrates instead.)
- Mezotrace, a calcium-magnesium source: four to six 1,200 milligram tablets daily
- Red clover (calcium-magnesium), available from herbal pharmacies or health-food stores
- Coenzyme Q_{10}, 400 to 600 milligrams

For complete information on the Lifestar Cancer Restoration Protocol, contact: Lifestar Millenium, Inc.; 2175 E. Francisco Blvd., #A-2; San Rafael, CA 94901; tel (415) 457-1400 or (800) 858-7477; fax (415) 457-8887.

fear of side effects. In the presence of cancer, for example, up to 1400 milligrams daily is not too much.
Unlike penicillin or other synthetic drugs, your body
will not become immune to the effects of lactoferrin,
because it's something your body is familiar with and
knows how to handle. If you're suffering with serious
illness, you should be working with a physician on a
complete treatment program.

For information on purchasing lactoferrin, see the
"Guide to Sources and Availability" on page 167.

Chapter 2

Infopeptides: The Next Generation Immune Booster

The Health Sciences Institute has been tracking the progress of a truly amazing natural product that has successfully treated everything from acute viral attacks to serious, chronic, and even life-threatening disorders. But until recently, this substance was available only to the small number of physicians involved in or aware of the research. We can finally share news of the healing potential of infopeptides, because an infopeptide product is now available to you.

On the basis of research done thus far, infopeptides have the potential to revolutionize at least three major areas of treatment:

(1) immune dysfunctions (from minor to major, including AIDS)
(2) childhood diarrhea
(3) myalgias and muscle pains, including arthritis and fibromyalgia

Recently, physicians at one of the most important and successful cancer centers in the world, Klinik St. George in Bad Aibling, Germany, became aware of this research. They are so impressed that they are using this product, along with lactoferrin (see Chapter 1) and the mushroom formula (see Chapter 3) to treat 100 cancer patients.

Biochemical research finds a previously unknown compound in colostrum

Infopeptides are a type of peptide found in milk and colostrum (the mother's "first milk") and were not previously known to exist. They are fundamentally different from colostrum and lactoferrin because they appear to have no direct antiviral or antibacterial properties of their own. They do, however, contain chemically coded instructions that appear to be vitally important to a properly regulated immune system.

Infopeptides, however, are not found naturally in breast milk. The longer peptide chains have to be broken down into shorter segments in order to work. This appears to happen naturally in the process of sucking milk from the breast — probably a result of a combination of physical manipulation and enzymes in the mouth of the newborn. Once they are activated in this way, infopeptides have an impressive ability to trigger powerful antiviral, antibacterial, and antiprotozoal immune functions. In that sense, their action is more hormone-like than nutrient-like. But they seem to be self-regulating in a way that artificial hormones are not. As noted by Staroscik, et al. in *Molecular Immunology* (vol. 210, no. 120, pp. 1277-82):

> [A] small-chain polyprotein-rich peptide in colostrum. . . has the same ability to regulate the activity of the immune system as the hormones of the thymus gland do. It activates an underactive immune system, helping it move into action against disease-causing organisms. It also

suppresses an overactive immune system, such as is often seen in the autoimmune diseases. [It] also appears to act on T cell precursors to produce helper T cells and suppressor T cells. The effect is similar to that of thymus hormones.

(Note: This country's most widely prescribed drug — synthetic estrogen — reduces the function of the thymus.)

Infopeptides are unique because of their ability to control both underactive and overactive immune systems (*Archives of Immunology & Therapeutic Experiments,* vol. 41, no. 5-6, 1993, pp. 275-9). Research has linked these polypeptides to widespread biological actions that alleviate inflammation, nervous disorders, and even sleep patterns (*Trends in Neuroscience,* vol. 18, no. 3, 1995, pp. 130-6).

Another exciting aspect of the infopeptide mode of action is that it is not dose-dependent. That is, once a very small amount of an infopeptide is consumed, an increased dose does nothing more.

Help for arthritis, fibromyalgia, AIDS, and more

"Cytolog" is the name given to infopeptide products developed by a company that has been studying infopeptides since 1992. In a small-scale study, 82 percent of rheumatoid arthritis patients experienced "good or very good" results within two to six weeks with the use of Cytolog. Subjects with osteoarthritis all reported "good or very good" responses; one patient is in complete remission. All of the patients had been taking at least one drug, and many of them had been taking up to four drugs — all to no avail. The participants had been suffering from six to 20 years.

Cytolog helped to fight acute (and potentially lethal) diarrhea in children in Guatemala. Worldwide, between 5 and 10 million children die every year from diarrhea. . . making the implications of this research profound.

In another as-yet-unpublished study, this one in Baltimore, AIDS patients showed a 50 percent reduction in symptoms in a short period of time with just 5 to 10 milliliters of Cytolog per day.

It will be months or even years before these findings appear in major medical journals, but because they are so significant, we are trying to get the word out as quickly as possible.

Doctors report incredible recoveries

Jeff Anderson, M.D., of Corte Madera, California, described his own experience with Cytolog after he contracted viral myalgic meningoencephalitis (a brain inflammation). He used two 5-milliliter doses per day for a week and found the results nothing short of amazing. He encountered rapid relief of inflammatory-connective-tissue pain (particularly myalgic pain and stiffness, as well as headache) within two or three minutes.

Dr. Arnold Takemoto, from Scottsdale, Arizona, stated that he thought the reports on Cytolog "too good to be true" when he first tested it clinically. He has been working with more than 500 active patients with medical problems that baffle traditional allopathic medicine. Dr. Takemoto's specialties are chronic fatigue immune-deficiency syndrome and fibromyalgia (two of the fastest-growing diseases among women), along with specialized consultation on referred patients with stage-4 cancer. Takemoto reports that his patients are experiencing incredible results with Cytolog.

Shingles, digestive problems, joint pain: All show dramatic improvement

Teresa E. Quinlin, M.D., of Winchester, Ohio, has seen dramatic improvement in acute viral illnesses, including shingles. Gastritis and other digestive problems have also been quickly resolved. One woman suffering from polymyalgia rheumatica (a painful disease of the collagen tissue) had a 90 percent reduction in joint and muscle pain. Dr. Quinlin hopes to see a total remission in this case.

Are cows good enough?

Is the bovine source just as good as the human derivation? The answer is probably yes. Bovine colostrum and lactoferrin are close but not precise matches to human counterparts. Certain infopeptides from cows, however, are believed to be 100 percent identical to those found in human milk.

For those who are lactose intolerant, it's also important to recognize that milk sugars responsible for lactose intolerance and the proteins responsible for cow's-milk allergies are largely absent in colostrum. Considering the small doses needed for effectiveness and the very small concentration of lactose remaining, the use of colostrum products should be of no concern to those with milk sensitivities.

Cytolog appears to be safe and well-tolerated when taken under a variety of circumstances and over extended periods of time. The benefits do not diminish but tend to increase over time. In fact, those who take Cytolog for three months or more relate that the benefits persist indefinitely even after they stop taking it.

We predict that you'll be hearing much more about infopeptides in the very near future. See the "Guide to Sources and Availability" on page 167.

Chapter 3

The Magic of Medicinal Mushrooms

Mushrooms grow in a hostile environment. They exist at the last rung of the food chain, living off fallen trees and decayed material, competing with bacteria and other environmental "lowlifes." In order for a mushroom spore to thrive, it must have an aggressive, proactive immune system, especially since mushrooms excrete their digestive enzymes outside of their cells. Their excretions must be able to immobilize the pathogens around them, so that the mushrooms can reabsorb the digested nutrients — uncontaminated — back into their cells.

It's no surprise, then, that fungi provide exceptionally powerful immune-system support — especially when compared with other plant medicines.

"Think of your immune system as an information bank," says David Law, biologist and co-founder of Gourmet Mushrooms in Sebastopol, California. "Every time your body has to cope with a foreign substance, your immune system protects you by expelling or killing the invader. It then stores the information so it can protect you against this kind of threat in the future. The mushroom has certain components that challenge your immune system without actually endangering you."

Each species of mushroom has a variety of active

compounds, such as glycoproteins, polysaccharides, enzymes, alkaloids, glycans, triterpenoids, nucleotides, and steroids. It is through the combinations of these compounds that certain mushrooms are believed to target the human immune system and aid in neuron transmission, metabolism, hormonal balance, and the transport of nutrients and oxygen.

The polysaccharides, for example, the large molecular-weight sugar molecules that have been studied since the 1950s for their antitumor and immunostimulating properties, resemble those found in bacteria. Specifically, the polysaccharides increase your production of macrophages and T cells. Macrophages are the "big-eater" cells that destroy foreign invaders, toxic chemicals, and tumor cells. T cells are those that have the remarkable ability to recognize chemical markers on virus-infected cells, yeast cells, and bacteria, targeting them for destruction.

Thus, the polysaccharides in a mushroom may "fool" your immune system into mounting an immune response, although the mushroom poses no actual threat.

An ongoing commitment to excellence

In order to offer the public the finest medicinal products possible, Malcolm Clark of Gourmet Mushrooms, Inc. seeks out only the strongest isolates and cultivates them via a patented process that he studied under Dr. Tsuneto Yoshii of the Yoshii Mycological Institute in Japan.

At least twice a year, Clark travels to remote areas in search of specimens to culture. It's not uncommon for him to camp out for days in a forest, observing a mushroom's response to various stimuli, so that he can duplicate the environment in his lab. It's this level of dedication, knowledge, and determination that has built Gourmet Mushrooms into the valuable medicinal-mushroom supplier it is today. In fact, it was Malcolm Clark who brought the first shiitake mushroom to North America more than 20 years ago!

Today, Gourmet Mushrooms grows more varieties of mushrooms than any other company in the world. Half the mushrooms cultured are medicinal "nutraceuticals." Through tight control and monitoring — from strain selection to the special cultural process — Gourmet Mushrooms consistently produces the highest-potency, highest-quality medicinal mushrooms.

A new preventive mushroom panacea

"Most people think they should take medicinal mushrooms in a crisis situation, such as in the presence of cancer or AIDS," says Law. "But you shouldn't wait. Cancer takes years to grow, and it can be slowed or stopped at any stage. Taking the mushrooms every day challenges and builds your immune system. . . to prepare you for whatever viruses, bacteria, or toxins come along."

Clark and Law have been working hard to develop the ideal daily mushroom supplement. The goal: to combine the most active strains for a preventive panacea that injects vitality into your immune system, stimulating every component into action. They've met that goal. The new product contains six different medicinal mushrooms plus a high-potency vitamin C supplement. The six mushrooms in this formula are Ganoderma lucidum (reishi), Lentinula edodes (shiitake), Cordyceps sinensis, Grifola frondosus (maitake), Coriolus versicolor, and Schizophyllum commune.

Containing the most powerful and well-documented immune-enhancing mushrooms known, this formula is unique. In fact, four of the mushrooms included — shiitake, C. versicolor, S. commune, and reishi — elicit such a powerful immune response that they're officially listed by the Japanese government as prescription-adjunct cancer therapies.

When used along with chemotherapy or radiation, these mushrooms (1) improve the effectiveness of traditional treatment, (2) increase remission and survival rates, and (3) help cancer patients maintain their health and well-being during chemotherapy by vigorously supporting the immune system. This is accomplished because white-blood-cell counts remain stable while symptoms like weight loss and nausea are minimized.

The Gourmet Mushrooms product contains only natural, unprocessed, unrefined constituents. This is important for two reasons. First, it ensures that you get the benefit of the synergy of the entire mushroom biomass. Second, the refined mushroom extracts may prove too strong to be used as a daily preventive. The Japanese preparations provide high doses of the refined mushroom extracts, but the fact is that a lower dosage may work better for prevention!

"Many times, we get sick because of imbalances in our systems that allow opportunistic pathogens to attack our bodies," explains David Law. "The key is to regulate these systems, not overload them. Most often, your whole body works on a feedback mechanism. If you don't have enough of something, your body will produce more. But if you have too much, your body will shut off production. A small dosage stimulates your body to do the work on its own."

Actions:
- Aids in neuron transmission, metabolism, hormonal balance, and the transport of nutrients and oxygen

Benefits:
- Strengthens the ability of the immune system to resist bacterial and viral infection
- Increases T cells that destroy foreign invaders

Gourmet Mushrooms, Inc. sells its products primarily to physicians, health-food stores, and pharmaceutical companies. For information on finding a distributor near you, see the "Guide to Sources and Availability" on page 167.

Chapter 4

Calcium Elenolate: Nature's Most Powerful Antibiotic

Tomorrow's #1 threat to your health . . . is here today

You may not believe it now, but infectious "smart bugs" are going to be the No. 1 threat to your health. In the past 15 years, death by infectious disease has already gone from being the fifth-leading killer in the United States to being the third-leading one!

And now, nine disease-causing bugs — bugs we thought we'd beaten long ago — have returned, stronger than the original strains. . . bringing a plague of dangerous and even deadly illnesses, including blood poisoning, tuberculosis, meningitis, pneumonia, sinusitis, gonorrhea, and bacteremia. Once, doctors could destroy these bacteria with powerful drugs. That was back in the golden age of antibiotics.

Today, it doesn't matter how quickly we invent drugs to kill them. Faster than we can create new antibiotics in our laboratories, deadly bacteria are developing resistance to the potent but limited drugs. There is one way, however, to stop these superbugs. We can outsmart them, using the tremendous protective power of nature.

Nature's most promising antibiotic, antiviral, and antifungal agent is a compound derived from the olive leaf, called calcium elenolate. As the number of drug-resistant superbugs continues to increase, so will the urgent need for olive-leaf extract.

This plant extract not only helps your body battle· the dangerous bugs that cause infectious disease but also detoxifies your entire system, enhances your energy, improves your circulation, activates key components of your immune system, and has beneficial effects on cholesterol and blood-sugar levels.

The history of calcium elenolate

Treatments made from the olive-leaf extract have been around for at least 150 years, with records dating back to 1827, when it was used as a treatment for malaria — with no side effects other than those produced by the ethanol wine used in these special ethanolic preparations. In 1906, the olive-leaf extract was reportedly far superior to quinine for the treatment of malaria, but quinine, because it was easier to administer, became the treatment of choice.

In 1957, the active ingredient of olive-leaf extract, oleuropein, was isolated and studied as a treatment for high blood pressure and other types of heart disease, again with no mention of toxic or other side effects. From 1970 to the present, a hydrolyzed form of oleuropein has been tested and found effective against dozens of different viruses and many strains of bacteria. None of these experiments noted any toxicity.

Now in tablet form, olive-leaf extract is making a comeback. From Mexico we have reports describing dramatic malaria remissions, but the therapeutic potential of the olive leaf is much more far-reaching. It's been proven to work in a number of specific ways:

- It **stunts the growth** of viruses or bacteria by interfering with certain amino-acid production processes necessary for those pathogens to grow.
- It **inhibits the spread** of the pathogen by preventing shedding, budding, or assembly at the cell membrane (i.e., it inactivates the virus or bacterium).
- It can enter your infected cells and **shut down viral replication** processes.
- In the case of retroviruses, such as HIV, it neutralizes the production of enzymes that are essential for a retrovirus to alter the RNA of a healthy cell.
- It **directly stimulates phagocytosis** — your immune system's ability to "eat" foreign microorganisms that don't belong in your body.

Clearly, this substance is highly complex — much more so than synthetic antibiotics — and this complexity is one of the keys to its success.

The importance of natural antibiotics in a dangerous age of infectious diseases

Independent research has shown that olive-leaf extract can be used as an adjunct treatment for influenza, meningitis, Epstein-Barr virus (EBV), encephalitis, the common cold, herpes I and II, HHV-6, HHV-7, shingles, HTLV-I, HTLV-II, HIV/ARC/AIDS, CFIDS, CMV, hepatitis B, pneumonia, sinusitis, tuberculosis, gonorrhea, malaria, bacteremia, urinary-tract infections, severe diarrhea, blood poisoning, and surgical infections.

Because it's a natural substance, olive-leaf extract has a much wider range of actions than man-made antibiotics. It contains a maze of chemicals — harmless to us — that lie in wait for invading bacteria. In this way, olive-leaf extract is very much like garlic, the traditional herbal cure-all. Garlic contains 17 amino acids, 33 sulfur compounds, plus copper, germanium, selenium, zinc, calcium, iron, potassium, magnesium, and vitamins A, B-1, and C-2. As you can imagine, it is much more difficult for an invading bacterium to develop resistance in the face of such a complex mixture of active chemicals.

Plant medicines like olive-leaf extract offer a great deal of promise for the future treatment of infectious diseases. According to experts at the Centers for Disease Control in Atlanta, medicine must continue to probe natural resources if it is to provide effective health care for all. Nature has evolved germ killers far more potent than any that laboratory scientists can invent. The olive-leaf extract is one of these germ killers.

Safety

In 1970, the Upjohn Pharmaceutical Company conducted and published a safety study on the use of olive-leaf extract in lab animals. An extrapolation of Upjohn's figures reveals that even at doses several hundred times the recommended amount, no toxic or other adverse side effects are likely to appear.

Bonus heart-health benefits of this special olive-leaf compound

The Mediterranean diet, rich in vegetables, fruits, grains, and olive oil, has recently been linked to a low incidence of heart disease. According to many studies, the olive-leaf compound has been found to serve as a vasodilator (it opens up your blood vessels), to prevent LDL oxidation (which causes hardened arteries), and even to help with diabetes and high blood pressure.

It thoroughly cleanses and detoxifies your system. In fact, the manufacturers of olive-leaf-extract supplements warn that you may experience significant detoxification symptoms. These symptoms — which can vary from stomach rumblings and other digestive disorders to mild headaches — are positive signs that the supplement is "at work." You can lessen these side effects, however, with a program of vitamin C supplementation, taken to bowel tolerance, and/or a probiotic formula to ensure strong, beneficial microflora in your bowel.

Generally, the recommended amount of olive-leaf extract is one or two 500-milligram tablets daily. After about two weeks, you can increase the amount to six or eight capsules daily. When you begin to feel better, reduce the amount to one or two capsules daily.

Actions:

- Halts growth and spread of bacteria, fungi, and viruses
- Prevents oxidation of LDL cholesterol
- Stimulates phagocytosis

Benefits:

- Detoxifies and cleanses
- Supports heart health
- Enhances circulation
- Supports the immune system
- Has beneficial effect on cholesterol and blood-sugar levels

---

Please turn to the "Guide to Sources and Availability" on page 167 for information on obtaining olive-leaf extract (calcium elenolate).

Section II

The Power of Panaceas

*U*nlike synthetic drugs, developed to produce a single chemical effect in the body, natural remedies are far more multifaceted, and they often have a multitude of beneficial effects. These so-called panaceas are among the most treasured of all natural healing agents, because they work by helping the body restore itself to proper balance and function.

In this chapter, you will learn about six substances from around the world that qualify as true panaceas. Each of them, through its own unique modes of action, can restore health and vitality, offering relief from a wide range of seemingly unrelated conditions. Put the power of a panacea to work for you.

Chapter 5

Garum Armoricum: The Ancient Panacea "With a Thousand Virtues"

In A.D. 43, Emperor Claudius' personal physician, Scribonius Largus, proclaimed it "the product with a thousand virtues." Largus brought this potent remedy back home from Armorica (today called Brittany). It was a remedy the likes of which the Romans had never seen: a powerful medicine made from a rare and unique deepwater fish. The Romans called it "garum," which translates today as "fish sauce."

Garum is a fermented, self-digested fish food made from very specific parts — including the brain and stomach — of a very specific fish: the great bluefish.

The Romans were astonished — and pleased — to discover that people who took garum enjoyed. . .

- renewed energy and strength (It was popular among soldiers!)
- reversal of painful, dragging illnesses, such as sinus pain and migraines
- bright moods and relief from depression

Garum was treasured among the ancients. It was

so valuable a commodity that ancient Europeans built hundreds of factories to produce and store this natural remedy, including one in western Spain with the capacity to store more than 2 million pounds of it. . . big business for the Romans!

Today, science has replaced the wooden vats and superstitions with machines and scientific knowledge. Now we understand that the ingredients mixed together in those vats were the building blocks your body needs to thrive. Today's version of garum is called garum armoricum, named for the place it was first discovered.

Health Sciences Institute panelists have been using garum to treat a wide range of symptoms, including. . . depression. . . fatigue. . . headaches. . . joint pain . . . chest pain. . . back pain. . . PMS. . . anxiety. . . and panic attacks. They report tremendous results after only days of treatment with garum.

Hundreds of years of clinical proof

The Romans didn't have controlled, double-blind tests. When something did *not* work, it quickly went the way of all flesh. But when a remedy *did* work, word of its success quickly spread. It's no wonder hundreds of garum factories have been discovered throughout modern-day Spain, Italy, North Africa, Belgium, England, and Austria. Archeologists have even excavated a well-preserved garum shop at Pompeii!

But today, the Western medical community demands — with good reason — that all new substances be tested with controlled, double-blind studies. Many countries around the world have put garum to the test. And it is passing with flying colors!

One French study tested 40 individuals suffering from symptoms of asthenia — meaning, literally, "without strength." Asthenia covers a range of chronic fatigue and depression disorders. The subjects took garum armoricum for 15 days, rating their symptoms before and after treatment, using the Asthenia Symptoms Index. The impressive results:

- sleep quality: 43% improvement
- mental fatigue: 44% improvement
- general well-being: 75% improvement
- speech problems: 33% improvement

Defeat your "deadliest" emotions

Anxiety, hostility, and stress are the most dangerous emotions in the world. In 1995, the American College of Family Practitioners reported that stress is an important component of at least 85 percent of the illnesses we face today, including heart disease and cancer. What's more, emotional stress and anxiety are also proven to. . .

- erode your immune system and damage delicate hormonal balances, such as those of the adrenal, pituitary, thyroid, and thymus glands
- increase your risk of getting a cold or infection by up to four times
- interfere with digestion, increase your heart rate and blood pressure, alter brain

chemistry, and affect your metabolic and immune functioning

One Japanese study specifically studied the stress-reducing, health-enhancing properties of garum. Researchers measured the ability of hospital patients to produce alpha waves with a biofeedback machine after treatment with garum amoricum. (Alpha waves increase when we're relaxed and decrease when we're under stress.)

After the subjects took garum for three months, their alpha wave scores had more than tripled — an effect surpassed only by prescription narcotic and psycholeptic drugs. But the critical difference is that garum has no side effects. And garum is powerful enough to balance even the most serious clinical depression. Patients experience fewer mood swings; less anxiety, agitation, and melancholia; improved feelings of well-being; diminished malaise; and better sleep quality. Improvements in physical energy and stamina are also frequently reported.

Garum is safe, nontoxic, nonaddictive, nonprescription, and free from side effects.

Why this unique fish is the most reliable source for these healing nutrients

Remarkably, the bluefish, unlike any other fish (the Romans tried others to no avail), has the precise combination of chemicals and nutrients your body needs to stabilize everything from your mood to your blood pressure.

One of the reasons garum nourishes and protects your heart is that, as a product of a fatty fish, it provides you with essential fatty acids that raise your good cholesterol and keep your blood unsticky. But, unlike regular fish-oil extract, it also delivers super-powerful antioxidants that protect you from free-radical damage. It also contains rich stores of amino acids, which are important for keeping your cells properly nourished, cleansed, energized, and protected from invading toxins.

Garum is a raw-food supplement containing bioactive ingredients, such as enzymes, that control virtually everything that happens in your body: breathing, eating, sleeping, dreaming, thinking, and even feeling. You can only get enzymes from raw, living organisms. The problem is, however, that you will probably never get enough of them from the typical American diet, since enzymes are so readily processed out of foods by cooking, storing, and freezing.

The fact that it's such a powerhouse of rare and essential nutrients could be one of the reasons garum is more effective than herbs and vitamins for pain relief. But garum also contains neuropeptides, which stimulate endorphins, your body's own homemade painkillers.

Mother Nature's most powerful opiate

Believe it or not, the same chemicals your body makes when you laugh, kiss, take a warm bath, or do anything else you love to do are potentially powerful enough to relieve chronic aches and pains — if you have the secret catalyst that gets them going.

Garum is that secret catalyst.

Garum contains powerful chemicals that kill pain naturally and make you feel good. These chemicals, which are strings of various combinations of amino acids, are called peptides. Some peptides act on your hormone production, some act on your brain cells, and some affect the way you feel.

Peptides that affect feelings of pain and pleasure are called endorphins. Endorphins can slow your breathing and lower your blood pressure. They exert a calming influence by blocking the transmission of pain signals in your brain. Because they can be as effective as morphine in certain circumstances, they have been called the body's own opiates. Endorphins are considered the "feel-good" substances that heighten one's sense of well-being. They are believed to play a critical role in promoting:

- a more positive attitude toward life
- enhanced alertness
- improved vitality

Your body naturally releases endorphins when you exercise. They are responsible for the euphoric feeling known as the "runner's high." Hypnosis and acupuncture may also liberate these natural painkillers, as does any pleasant emotional experience.

Since garum is a source of pure, "raw" peptides, it is clear to see why it has such a powerful relaxing and pain-relieving effect!

Actions:
- Provides high-quality nutrients, including all eight essential amino acids, essential fatty acids, antioxidants, peptides, and bioactive raw food enzymes

Benefits:
- Provides peptides; helps breathing and blood pressure
- Supplies antioxidants and essential fatty acids to support heart health and circulation
- Provides amino acids to nourish and support cells
- Produces overall mood-boosting effects
- Offers emotional-stress relief
- Helps with stress-induced symptoms, including back pain, headaches, eating disorders, frequent colds, insomnia, premenstrual tension, and more

The recommended amount of garum armoricum is generally two to four 200-milligram capsules daily while symptoms are present. When symptoms have disappeared, the amount may be gradually cut down and finally discontinued. For purchasing information, see the "Guide to Sources and Availability" on page 167.

Chapter 6

Organic Germanium: "Electrify" Your Health

Supercharged mineral discovered! In 1886, a German chemist discovered an unidentified chemical — a mineral occurring in small quantities in foods, coal deposits, and the earth's crust. He called the substance "germanium." In 1950, Dr. Kazuhiko Asai, a brilliant Japanese chemist, discovered traces of germanium in fossilized plants. The next news about germanium came from Russia, where reports suggested that it had anticancer properties.

A few years later, Dr. Asai discovered that many healing plants — such as garlic, aloe, comfrey, chlorella, ginseng, shiitake mushrooms, and watercress — have significant concentrations of germanium. The holy water of Lourdes, known for its therapeutic value, also contains germanium.

In 1967, Dr. Asai managed to synthesize a new compound of germanium and found that the manufactured substance also had amazing curative abilities! This product has come to be known as "organic germanium." (You may wonder how something man-made can be called "organic." The reason is that anything containing carbon in its molecular architecture is organic. Thus, synthetically derived germanium is, according to definition, organic.)

How does germanium "electrify" your health?

If you are old enough to have assembled a crystal radio in your youth, you may remember the germanium diode crystal, which was responsible for bringing in the radio signal that you heard in your earphone. The germanium atom is so structured that it accepts and transmits electrons, giving it a semiconductor capability. This means it becomes an electrostimulator, inducing the flow of electricity. In its pure metallic form, germanium is used extensively in the electronics industry for transistors, fiber optics, and other diverse applications.

Biologically, it appears to be able to stimulate electrical impulses on a cellular level. Science has established — as undisputed fact — that our bodies, our nerves, and our muscles are all electrically linked. So any substance that can enhance our electrical "connections" is bound to have a profound and life-giving effect.

Germanium has several unique and extremely valuable properties. It acts as:

- **an oxygen enhancer:** It has been shown to increase the flow of oxygen to all cells, especially in those areas that suffer from poor circulation.
- **a detoxifier:** Because of its chemical structure, germanium tends to bind or chelate (grab) and then remove toxic compounds and harmful substances from your system.

- **an adaptogen:** It "normalizes" your body's functions and adjusts to your specific needs. In the case of cancer, for example, it doesn't kill the cancer cells directly but stimulates your immune defenses to produce the substance that will, in turn, help to destroy the antagonist.
- **an immune catalyst:** Germanium helps to convert inactive macrophages — important immune cells — to active cells. It also enhances interferon production and increases natural killer cells.
- **a brain booster:** It has been reported to increase mental capacity, possibly because it helps your body send oxygen to the delicate tissues of the brain.

But even after 20 years of clinical and lab research, germanium is still virtually unknown in the United States. It remains a "mysterious" healing substance. Unfortunately, it takes many years from the time a discovery is recognized to the time when its importance is truly understood and accepted. In fact, medical historians inform us that the average delay from journal reporting to actual clinical use can be 50 or more years!

Ironically, the better a substance works. . .the more difficult it is to convince the mainstream medical community of its value. If a manufacturer wants the FDA to evaluate germanium and approve it for specific usage, it will have to show precisely how it works. But germanium appears to have endless curative abilities. Even if we had the technology and know-how to explain its various actions, it could still take decades to prove each application to the FDA.

Actions:

- Binds to toxins and metals so that they are easily removed
- Increases oxygen flow and uptake throughout your body
- Enhances interferon production
- Normalizes and balances bodily functions like blood pressure and immune-system activity

Benefits:

- Promotes quick healing through better circulation
- Promotes quick pain relief
- Helps prevent circulation problems
- Boosts energy and mood

Nevertheless, germanium works. And you can use it today! For prevention, one 150-milligram capsule daily is generally recommended. In the presence of serious illness, physicians often recommend from 500 to 2,000 milligrams (2 grams) daily. Some manufacturers supply germanium by the kilo, at a substantial savings. For purchasing information, see the "Guide to Sources and Availability" on page 167.

Chapter 7

Noni: The Polynesian Wonder-Worker

The noni plant (also known as "nano," "nonu," and even "nono") is classified as morinda citrifolia and has been used by Tahitians, Hawaiians, and other Polynesians for medicinal purposes for as long as those cultures have been in the South Seas. Native names for the tree include the "Headache Tree" and the "Pain-killer Plant." Also called "Indian Mulberry," it's a small, wandering evergreen found in tropical coastal regions and forest areas up to 1,300 feet above sea level.[1]

A traditional defender of good health, noni is Hawaii's second most frequently prescribed medicinal plant today. It's no surprise, then, that Hawaiian literature and lore chronicle endless accounts of noni's virtues — reports that range from the anecdotal to the scientific.

The Department of Pharmacology and Pathology at the University of Hawaii has documented the anti-cancer activity of noni on test animals. In one experiment, it significantly prolonged the life of mice with implanted lung carcinoma cells. The researchers theorized that noni works by stimulating the activity of T cells within the immune system, which helps to explain why it is used successfully for such a wide range of illnesses.

1 Morton, J.F., "The Ocean-Going Noni, or Indian Mulberrry, and Some of its Colorful Relatives," in *Economic Botany*, 1992.

Researchers note that noni can also be helpful in cases of hypertension, diabetes, and arthritis. It can be invaluable as an adjunct treatment with chemotherapy.[2] Hawaiians were (and still are) using noni for the lassitude of old age.[3] So here we have a product that can fight a bevy of formidable degenerative diseases, minimize the miserable side effects of chemotherapy, and even offer a shot in the arm for the fatigue problems of old age.

And there's more! According to the long list of testimonials from users of the Tahitian variety, noni juice is an effective treatment for arthritis, premenstrual cramps, gastric ulcers, sprains, poor digestion, breast cancer, and eye problems. It has even been shown to be beneficial for carpal tunnel syndrome. And it's fast-acting, too! Users have reported nearly overnight cures for a multitude of serious long-term illnesses.

Some of these benefits can be explained by several specific actions, observed in laboratory tests: Noni appears to exhibit a smooth muscle stimulatory effect, anti-microbial activity, as well as analgesic (pain-relieving) and tranquilizing properties.

Noni: a medicinal food used the world over

The noni plant is often found growing along lava flows, accounting for its abundance on Hawaii and other volcanic islands. It grows easily and requires little care. But, left largely uncultivated, noni was becoming scarce in the mid '80s. Now that its medicinal prop-

2 *Proceedings of Western Pharmacology*, vol. 37, 1994, pp. 145-6.
3 *Hawaiian Medical Journal*, vol. 25, no. 3, 1966, pp. 223-30.

erties are being recognized, however, the noni tree is enjoying a resurgence in the islands.

In India, Java, and Africa, different parts of the plant are used for various medical applications. The fruit, for example, relieves diarrhea; the bark mitigates stomach complaints; and the flower is good for conjunctivitis. In the Caribbean, the leaves are poulticed on wounds and rheumatic joints and are applied on the head to relieve pain. In Guam, the juice is squeezed from the flowers and applied to sore eyes; the fruit pulp is used as an insecticidal shampoo.

Another melding of an ancient cure with today's high technology

Several multilevel marketing companies promote both Tahitian and Hawaiian varieties of noni, packaged as liquid juice extracts and as powdered whole fruits. But the Health Sciences Institute has identified one source, not yet widely known or promoted, with a unique way of producing noni products.

In this process, Hawaiian-grown noni is freeze-dried, using the entire fruit, not just the juice. (Freeze-drying provides a more concentrated product and is one of the safest forms of preservation.) After freeze-drying, a colloidal extraction is produced, which can then be prepared in liquid or powder form. Colloids are more bioavailable because of their small particle size. They are also more stable. This colloidal noni product has been developed with the use of a break-through electro-colloidal, or nonchemical, proprietary process. In addition, unlike some other noni products, it does not have to be pasteurized and does not ferment.

For prevention, noni is taken once a day, preferably between meals, with amounts varying depending on the product. Polynesian folk tradition dictates that it be taken at a restful or peaceful time of day. For therapy, the amount can be increased. As with any natural tonic, noni can be used safely for nutritional and systemic support along with other pharmaceutical therapies. Of course, if you use prescription drugs, you should always discuss with your doctor any supplements you are taking. See page 167 for the "Guide to Sources and Availability."

Chapter 8

Emu Oil: Nourish Your Skin and Relieve Muscle and Joint Pain

The emu (or Dromaius novaehollandiae) is the second-largest bird (the ostrich is number one); an adult typically stands 5 feet tall, weighs 120 pounds, and is able to run 30 miles an hour. An ancient species, it's believed to be as much as 80 million years old, co-existing with dinosaurs up until their demise about 65 million years ago. It's the only surviving species of its family, having weathered an attempt by Australian farmers to exterminate the emu population in the 1930s. Other species in Australia and Tasmania were not so lucky: we'll never be able to study the therapeutic assets of oils from the elephant bird or the moa.

Oil of emu — a skin panacea

For thousands of years, desert-dwelling Australians have been healing wounds and soothing painful joints with emu oil. Traditional applications of emu fat or oil also address a wide range of skin problems — a critical branch of aboriginal medicine, considering the harsh environment of the Australian outback. The oil has been used as a remedy for burns, wounds, and insect bites and as a sunscreen and moisturizer. Modern research on the properties of emu oil did not begin until the 1980s. As a result of the involvement of major Australian pharmaceutical companies at that time, emu oil products are now widely available in Australia where they're sold for use as massage oils, liniments, and lubricants.

Clinical studies corroborate the traditional uses of emu oil. Here is a summary of the findings by Dr. G.R. Hobday after 10 years of experience treating over 500 patients in Australia, without a single reported allergic reaction:

- **Burns:** promotes faster healing; lessens pain and scarring
- **Bruising and muscle aches:** reduces pain; shows anti-inflammatory action when massaged into strained muscles following exercise
- **Eczema:** diminishes irritation and inflammation of the skin
- **Joint pain:** reduces pain, swelling, and stiffness when a joint problem is close to skin
- **Keloids:** decreases scarring; has anti-inflammatory action against formation of keloid tissue (A keloid is irregular scar tissue forming on skin after trauma.)
- **Psoriasis:** shows limited benefit in some patients (Worth a try, isn't it?)
- **Wounds:** reduces scar tissue; has anti-inflammatory action on post-surgical wounds

Another clinical study now in progress at the Texas Tech University Health Sciences Center is suggesting similar results in the area of wound healing.

Emu oil is relatively high in both linoleic acid and linolenic acid, the two essential polyunsaturated fatty acids. "Essential" means it cannot be synthesized by your body, so it must be included in your diet. Linoleic and linolenic are the two EFAs (essential fatty acids) responsible for fish oil's importance in cardiac and vascular health. However, we should not fall into the trap of the reductionist approach. If these two EFAs were the only factors responsible for emu oil's thera-peutic properties, it would be easy to produce a fully effective synthetic substitute. But more than 25 differ-ent fatty acids have been isolated from various samples of emu oil. For example, it contains significant amounts of oleic acid, a known enhancer for the transport of bioactive compounds through the skin.

Arthritis, bursitis, and tendinitis begone!

A study conducted by Dr. Thom Leahey in 1995 found that emu-oil users reported significant reduc-tion of arthritic pain in their hands, while placebo par-ticipants were not as successful. Testimonials even include reports of relief for bursitis and tendonitis.

Dr. Michael Holick, professor of dermatology at Boston University, concluded that the growth of skin and hair is very much enhanced with the application of emu oil. "The hair follicles were more robust, the skin thickness was remarkably increased. . . Also, we discovered in the same test that over 80 percent of hair follicles that had been 'asleep' were awakened and began growing hair," reported Holick.

He also suggests, in an article in the *Drug and Cosmetics Industry* journal, that the sunscreen properties of emu derive from its ability to "lock down UVA/UVB absorbents more firmly to the skin and therefore increase the longevity of the sun-protection properties."

Emu oil is easily absorbed and transported through the fatty tissue of your skin, making it an excellent vehicle for delivering other therapeutic substances via topical application. Furthermore, it's non-comodogenic, which means it doesn't clog pores, even on the most sensitive skin — a common problem among oil products. So watch for emu oil as a base ingredient in a wide range of topically applied products that will no doubt flood the market in a short time!

Emu-oil products are reported to be in widespread use by major athletic teams, where they may help with various stress injuries. The oil seems to have many of the advantages of anti-inflammatory steroid drugs like cortisone. And because it works by activating natural healing and protective mechanisms, it lacks the devastating side effects of artificial steroids.

But new ideas move slowly through our mainstream medical community. It's likely that the coach of your favorite professional team (because of the oil's benefits for sprains and strains), or your veterinarian (because it has a long history of success with animals) will become familiar with the uses of emu oil long before your physician does. You should be aware of the large body of impressive information accumulating in support of emu oil for wound recovery and relief of muscle and joint pain.

Actions:
- Blocks UVA and UVB rays
- Has anti-inflammatory properties
- Reduces pain
- Stimulates hair follicles

Benefits:
- Lessens pain from burns, bruising, muscle aches, and joint pain
- Promotes faster healing of skin wounds
- Reduces formation of scar tissue
- Appears to increase hair growth

Because of its inherent safety and extraordinary effectiveness, emu oil should find an important place in your medicine cabinet. You'll discover applications for many common ailments because it can be used freely without fear of negative side effects. See the "Guide to Sources and Availability" on page 167 for information on obtaining emu oil.

Chapter 9

Natural Progesterone Cream: Restore Optimum Hormone Levels

Since World War II, our world has become a hormonal minefield

In the past 50 years, the world has been swamped with dangerous chemicals that we now know have serious health consequences for all of us. Many of these substances are "endocrine disrupters" — they disrupt the body's natural hormone balance by imitating the action of the natural hormone estrogen.

You can't avoid this chemical poisoning — the chemicals are simply too widespread. Some are commonly used in pesticides, fungicides, and insecticides; others show up in industrial chemicals, detergents, and food dyes. For example, red dye No. 3, added to hot dogs and other popular processed foods, emits an estrogen mimic.

Synthetic hormones are also created as byproducts in the manufacture of such everyday items as paper and plastics — the very plastics in which you may store your vitamins and wrap your foods; the plastics you sit on, cook with, eat with, and sleep on! The plastic

coating in a single can of peas contains a powerful estrogen mimic, the action of which is 300 million times
higher than the natural action of estradiol (the most
potent form of estrogen).

Your body, mistaking the synthetic estrogens all
around you for the real thing, accepts and processes
them, day in and day out, until your hormone balance
is thrown completely out of whack and your body is
dangerously overloaded with unnatural sex hormones.

Attention, men: Estrogen isn't just a female hormone. Men produce it too, and, believe it or not, too
much estrogen, whether you manufacture it or get it
from the environment, increases your risk of prostate
enlargement — just as too much testosterone has been
implicated as one of the causes of prostate cancer.

Environmental estrogen may be the cause of many modern ills

Dozens of studies in the past few years have led
researchers to the same conclusion: These chemicals
lower sperm counts and contribute to the sharp increases in testicular and prostate cancer, as well as
breast cancer and endometriosis. Rates of testicular
cancer have doubled, tripled, and even quadrupled in
some parts of the world in the last half of this century.
Breast-cancer rates have increased by over 30 percent
and prostate-cancer rates by 60 percent. Once a rare
disease, endometriosis (a painful inflammation of the
uterus that can cause sterility) now afflicts millions
of women.

Incidence of abnormal pregnancy is on the rise. Average sperm counts worldwide have decreased by 50 percent in the past 50 years. Many researchers believe that the widespread exposure to estrogen disrupters in the fetal stage 50 years ago contributed to our current high rates of infertility and sex-organ cancers. HSI panel members believe that lifetime exposure to estrogen mimics is a major cause of this epidemic of hormone-related diseases and disorders. You can't avoid these chemicals, but you can defend your body against their damaging effects.

You can rebalance your hormone ratios

The phenomenal success of natural progesterone therapy has been documented and validated over and over again. Don't confuse this with prescribed synthetic progestins. We are referring to cream-based products that contain a blend of wild Mexican yam (which has progesterone-type activity), a small amount of natural progesterone, and synergistic herbs. This combination appears to provide optimal benefit without the hazards associated with other popular hormone therapies.

Progesterone also favors the development of T cells in both men and women, thereby boosting immunity. It increases dopamine release, supplying a good precursor for adrenal hormones — again, for both sexes. Progesterone is a primary hormone responsible for the manufacture of other hormones, including cortisone. Cortisone works to reduce inflammation and suppress unwanted immune-system responses. This means that it can help with arthritis pain. It also has the overall effect of helping your body deal with stressful psychological situations.

Progesterone cream can relieve arthritis pain

When you supply your body with adequate amounts of progesterone, you may be able to restore cortisone levels to normal and to reduce — even eliminate — arthritic inflammation. Helpful for both rheumatoid arthritis and osteoarthritis, the most effective progesterone products contain a small amount of this hormone plus a few herbs with progesterone-type activity, including the now famous Mexican wild yam.

Protects against osteoporosis — in both men and women

In both men and women, progesterone protects against osteoporosis by working directly on cells called osteoblasts, which actually build new bone.

Keep in mind that estrogen therapy does not reverse osteoporosis. It merely reduces the rate of bone loss by affecting the activity of osteoclasts, the cells that cause calcium to leach out of your bones and re-enter your blood plasma. And if the estrogen is synthetic, the reduction in bone loss is only temporary.

Again and again, it's been demonstrated that after six months to a year of natural progesterone use, bone density can be increased even in women who are 70 and over.

A Revolutionary Fertility Indicator

One of the pleasures of reaching menopause is freedom from fear of pregnancy. But as women approach this rite of passage, it's often difficult to determine precisely when ovulation stops. Menstrual cycles become irregular in the later premenopausal years and may or may not necessarily be accompanied by ovulation. And even a remote chance of pregnancy is more than most premenopausal women want to worry about.

It's well-known that your saliva, viewed under a microscope, can be an instant and very accurate indicator of fertility. Now you can be your own lab technician. A newly introduced portable device allows anyone to get a microscopic glimpse of the particular crystalline structure that appears in the saliva when a woman is ovulating — without benefit of a medical laboratory. You just lick this optically enhanced slide, let it dry, and observe the results. It's ready to use again after rinsing with water. The source company, Personal Fertility Technologies, has prepared an instructional video and other materials to help interpret your results.

This is terrific technology put to great use — your peace of mind. You can get more information by contacting Personal Fertility Technologies directly at 11230 Gold Express Drive, Suite 310-272; Gold River, CA 95670; tel (888) 573-8123; fax (916) 944-4035.

An alternative to hormone replacement therapy

The dangers of the conventional practice of prescribing synthetic hormone replacement therapy for women are far more serious than generally recognized. Furthermore, the effectiveness of such therapy for reducing heart disease and osteoporosis has been seriously questioned.

A natural formula containing progesterone and herbs has the potential to relieve PMS and menopausal symptoms, including irritability, hot flashes, water retention, vaginal dryness, fatigue, and mood swings and help to protect against breast cancer, fibrocysts, and endometriosis. It also supports thyroid hormone actions, normalizes zinc and copper levels, normalizes blood clotting and blood-sugar levels, helps use fat for energy, and, according to endless anecdotal reports, may even restore lost libido.

A good formula for women should contain herbs like chamomile, burdock root, black cohosh, and Siberian ginseng — in addition to wild yam extract, a small amount of natural progesterone, and special oils to facilitate absorption and even moisturize the skin. The application of such a cream, when properly formulated, has been shown to play an important role in hormonal balance.

As Health Sciences Institute panel member Dr. Jesse Hanley points out, "The need for hormones suggests a hormone imbalance, which does not occur in isolation. That is, a hormone imbalance suggests a decline in other systems as well. That's why I prefer, when using hormone therapy, to add other stabilizing agents like herbs."

A progesterone preparation designed specifically for men

HSI panelist Dr. Howard Bezoza has tried administering testosterone therapy to men and has concluded that "believe it or not, testosterone therapy doesn't even raise hormonal levels. I've tried it with many men — in oral capsules, cream, and patches. And it creates a symphony of problems. Where most doctors go wrong is in measuring the single androgen (testosterone) and not measuring the whole picture. They miss the boat. There are too many other factors. Often these men have lower levels of other hormones as well, hormones like pregnenolone, DHEA, and estrogens that increase the risk of prostate problems."

A special men's formula containing progesterone and synergistic herbs has the potential to improve sperm quality and quantity and boost potency. It may shrink enlarged prostates and may protect against prostate and testicular cancer as well. Herbs that support male health, and also appear to work synergistically with progesterone, include Siberian ginseng, saw palmetto, wild oat straw, damiana, Ginkgo biloba, and gotu kola.

A little progesterone goes a long way!

In the case of hormones, more is not always better. In fact, you need only a small amount of progest-

Actions:

- Provides building blocks for other hormones
- Helps maintain optimum hormone balance in repro-
  ductive and sex-related organs
- May favor the development of T cells in both men
  and women

Benefits:

- Reduces the risks associated with estrogen overload
- Increases energy
- Normalizes libido
- Stabilizes mood
- Relieves depression
- Helps the body use fat for energy
- Boosts immunity
- Alleviates inflammation and pain
- Protects against osteoporosis by facilitating new bone
  growth

erone to get the desired results. If you're using one of
the high-dose preparations (some have as much as 900
or more milligrams of progesterone in a 2-ounce jar),
it is advisable to be under a doctor's care. You need to
be monitored periodically to be sure that you are not
getting too much of a good thing! Recent laboratory
results indicate that high doses of progesterone can lead
to an accumulation of hormones in your tissues.

The lower-dose preparations — usually 10 milligrams per 2-ounce jar — are safer, and they are just as
effective for most men and women when prepared with
the synergistic herbs described above. Recommended
usage of the low-dose cream is one-eighth to one-half

teaspoon a day. A 2-ounce jar should last one to two months. For purchasing information, see page 167 for the "Guide to Sources and Availability."

Do your cholesterol levels increase your risk of impotence?

Research from a Massachusetts male aging study shows that middle-aged and older men with low levels of HDL cholesterol are more likely to become impotent than men with high levels of HDL cholesterol. This is good news for two reasons:

(1) Contrary to popular beliefs, we know that impotence is not necessarily a function of aging.

(2) Men do have control over their HDL levels.

Many substances can lower LDL cholesterol (the bad cholesterol contributing to hardened arteries), but there's only one food that's known to raise HDL cholesterol. It's grape-seed oil, and it takes just 1 ounce daily to get the benefits.

The best grape-seed oil, Salute Sante, is available in health and gourmet shops. Salute Sante is superior because it is the only grape-seed oil processed at a low temperature, produced monthly (the UV-protected bottles are dated), and, unlike any other grape-seed oil in the marketplace, it retains natural chlorophyll. One supplier is Food and Vine, Inc.; 301 Poplar Ave., Suite 6; Mill Valley, CA 94941; tel (415) 388-8892.

Chapter 10

Probiotics: Help for the Postantibiotic Age

During World War II, a new wonder drug emerged: It was penicillin, the very first antibiotic. Today, "antibiotic" is a household word. It literally means "destructive of life," and the term is generally applied to substances that can kill or inhibit the growth of undesirable microorganisms. Now, of course, we know the sad truth: Antibiotics also annihilate beneficial microorganisms.

Probiotics are food supplements that encourage the growth and proliferation of the microorganisms that you want to have inside your body. (Probiotic means "promoting life.") Probiotic supplements, such as acidophilus, are now common, and for good reason. Average adults have several thousand billion bacteria in their digestive tracts — adding up to about 4 pounds of living material. Approximately 400 different species are represented. This complex mass of life forms, an entire ecosystem in miniature, is so vital to health that it's often thought of as an organ in its own right.

You probably know that these "good" bacteria help with digestion and elimination. If you're informed and health-conscious, you also know that they contribute vitamins, enzymes, and specialized, natural antibiotics and are also responsible for very specific functions in digestion and disease resistance.

Do we really need a probiotic?

If we ate nothing but fresh, raw, natural foods (uncorrupted by heat, preservatives, additives, or pesticides) and lived in a clean, unpolluted environment, would supplementation of our natural supply of intestinal microorganisms be necessary? The study of food history reveals that most traditional societies have included cultured food products as an important part of their diet. Yogurt, kefir, sauerkraut, fermented millet, fermented vegetables, tempeh, miso, and pickles have been embraced as offering health benefits for millennia.

Today, the commercial versions of virtually all of these foods are almost totally lacking in viable organisms. The bacteria that caused the fermentation of the food — the ones that we want in our intestinal tracts — are no longer capable of multiplying into the billions of living microorganisms required for optimal health. Even commercial yogurts, with only a few exceptions, don't supply sufficient live-organism counts.

In addition to lacking a good food source for favorable intestinal organisms, it's much more difficult for us to maintain intestinal flora when it is established. Poor diet, preservatives, additives, and pesticide residues are directly responsible. Antibiotic drugs are particularly damaging to intestinal bacteria, the effects lasting for weeks after the drugs are discontinued. So we turn to probiotic supplements. There are difficulties, however. This type of supplement is hard to produce accurately: the strains of the bacteria in a final product are often not the same as those intended — often one bacterial strain can negate another. Some strains may also have low potency and a short shelf life.

Freeze-drying presents problems because it essentially "boils" the water away under very low pressure, causing damage to cell membranes and other structures. This makes it impossible for microorganisms to proliferate when they are rehydrated. The most serious issue with many available probiotic supplements is the question of viability and potency after storage. Microorganisms tend to be very fragile and heat-sensitive, and their shelf life is typically only six months—under ideal conditions. Labeling laws do not address these factors, and few manufacturers will guarantee the performance of their products when measured on these terms.

One exception is a probiotic called "ProTec." The manufacturer guarantees it to have a potency of 1 billion live organisms per gram for three years after the date of packaging, with no refrigeration. (Now that's shelf life!) Even though ProTec has a lower potency than some probiotics, the effectiveness of this product appears to be superior because of the exceptionally high viability after years of storage.

Special attention has also been given to the specific strains of bacteria used. ProTec contains four species, grown in such a way as to prevent one strain from competing with another. The strains are literally "grown" together by means of a unique and proprietary process.

The following bacterial strains are used in ProTec:

(1) *Lactobacillus acidophilus.* The most common microorganism in the small intestine, it digests carbohydrates and produces lactase to digest milk sugar and lactic acid, thereby suppressing undesirable bacteria and yeast.

(2) *Lactobacillus casei.* Viable at a wider pH and temperature range than acidophilus, this strain performs many of the same functions when conditions are unfavorable to the proliferation of lactobacillus acidophilus.

(3) *Bifido bacterium bifidum.* This makes up the bulk of microorganisms in the large intestine, and nearly all of the intestinal flora in breast-fed infants. It produces a number of acids that appear to protect against undesirable bacteria, yeasts, and viruses. Highly susceptible to environmental stress, it declines significantly as people age.

(4) *Streptococcus faecium.* This fiber-loving bacterium may be involved in releasing lignans, substances that appear to have antitumor properties.

In contrast to most other powdered probiotic supplements, ProTec is not freeze-dried. The microorganisms are preserved by drying under mild heat, a carefully tuned process that puts these friendly bacteria in a state of suspended animation until they arrive in your intestines. It is designed to survive the acidic stomach environment and become activated by the alkaline environment of your intestines. To find sources for probiotics, refer to the "Guide to Sources and Availability" on page 167.

Section III

Breakthrough Solutions and Underground Cures

*N*ature supplies us with many potent and non-toxic solutions to the illnesses and conditions that we struggle with every day. At the Health Sciences Institute, we dedicate our resources to uncovering and researching the best of these solutions, and getting that information into your hands. If you are among the millions who live with high blood pressure, arthritis, depression, herpes, or other chronic conditions—and have felt let down by the "solutions" that traditional medicine has to offer—you'll find both help and hope in the pages that follow.

Chapter 11

Collagen Hydrolysate: Help Your Body Build New Cartilage

Arthritis is America's No. 1 disease. If you've tried conventional medicine, you know the truth: Drug therapy doesn't free you from pain and doesn't help to slow down your disease. What you may not know is that all conventional arthritis drugs — from NSAIDs (nonsteroidal anti-inflammatories) to steroids — carry serious risks to your health, both immediate and long-term.

The good news is that you no longer have to settle for conventional therapy. We've learned about a revolutionary treatment for joint care that relieves pain, can be used safely over the long term, and may actually help prevent joint problems. Only recently available in the United States, it has just been patented as a treatment for arthritis.

Tests for safety and effectiveness in lab animals, as well as clinical studies with humans suffering from all forms of arthritis, have been so successful that the FDA has approved a large-scale study on humans. Research suggests that in addition to relieving pain and restoring flexibility, it may actually help cartilage regrow. . . something that until now was believed impossible! This is no small feat. Unlike your liver or your heart, which can recover from devastating trauma, cartilage cannot heal itself. Once it's gone, it's gone (or so we thought).

A warning to all men and women over 35: You are losing your cartilage, little by little

Over time, the cartilage between your joints wears thin. Most doctors consider this wear and tear normal and inevitable. By the time you turn 35, you can be sure some measurable change in the shape of your cartilage has occurred. Almost everyone suffers from degenerative changes by that age. If you're over 55, your doctor probably expects to discover at least some symptoms of osteoarthritis.

There are two kinds of arthritis: You do NOT have to suffer from either

Rheumatoid arthritis is a chronic, inflammatory disorder that causes stiffness, deformity, and pain in joints and muscles — usually those of hands and feet, particularly knuckle and toe joints. Your joints gradually become inflamed and swollen, leading to the destruction of tissue and, in severe cases, deformity.

Unlike osteoarthritis, which progresses steadily over time, rheumatoid arthritis is a waxing/waning condition. You could have a single attack, or you might suffer several episodes that could leave you increasingly disabled. Rheumatoid arthritis is also associated with damage to the lungs, heart, nerves, and eyes. It's seen mostly in those between the ages of 40 and 60, but it can also affect children and teen-agers. Three times more women than men are afflicted. The causes are not fully understood, but it's considered an auto-immune problem: Immune-system defenders attack the joint tissues as if they were threats to your body.

Osteoarthritis is very different. It's the gradual wearing away of cartilage in your joints, generally considered a process of aging. As cartilage wears thin, your joint mobility decreases. Eventually, cartilage wears through completely. Whenever you flex your joints, your bones rub against one another, causing inflammation of the synovial tissues, which cushion the joints. Movement becomes difficult and painful.

The cause? If you ask mainstream doctors, most will tell you the cause is unknown. That's the traditional stance of the Arthritis Foundation and the orthodox medical community. The standard solution? Drugs: over-the-counter pain relievers, anti-inflammatory drugs, NSAIDs, cortisone-type drugs (steroids), gold salts, and even experimental cytotoxic (cell-killing) drugs.

NSAIDs are by far the most common therapy for arthritis. If you use NSAIDs, such as ibuprofen (Motrin), naproxen (Naprosyn), oxaprozin (Daypro), nabumetone (Relafen), or diclofenac (Voltaren), you should be aware that every year almost 25,000 people using these drugs suffer serious gastrointestinal side effects, including bleeding, ulceration, and perforation.

NSAIDs also interact with blood-pressure medicine. New evidence shows their long-term use can cause liver and kidney damage. They also may accelerate the destructive nature of arthritis. These effects can occur at any time, with or without warning symptoms. Your risk increases with longer use or higher dosages.

Then there are steroids — powerful drugs that present a host of serious health risks. To quote former Oriole baseball pitcher Jim Palmer, "Cortisone is a miracle drug. . . for a week!" By suppressing your immune-system response, steroids lessen swelling, soreness, and allergic reactions. In some cases, they give your body a chance to heal itself, but in the case of arthritis, they provide little more than a temporary fix.

Warning: Steroids are strong medicines and can have very serious side effects. Since they suppress your immune system, they can lower your resistance to infections and make them harder to treat. Steroids are broad-spectrum, which means they scatter their immune-suppressing effects throughout your body — from your liver to your central nervous system. Side effects of short-term use include frequent urination, mental depression, and sudden blindness. Side effects from long-term use can include insomnia, an increase in hair growth on the body and face, an irregular heartbeat, shortness of breath, and sudden death.

Even with all of these risks, neither NSAIDs nor steroids alter the arthritis process itself. And if they don't work, surgery is usually the final option: removal of badly inflamed joint synovia, joint realignment and reconstruction, tendon repair, joint fusion, or artificial joint replacement.

You can avoid this downward spiral of dangerous drugs and risky procedures

In Chapter 9, we discussed the effectiveness of natural progesterone cream for relieving arthritis pain and stiffness. Although natural progesterone therapy is much more effective than conventional drug therapy and is quite safe, it cannot restore worn-down cartilage. But one substance may actually help your body create *new* cartilage.

In European medical literature, the appearance of a therapeutic substance derived from collagen (cartilage protein) dates back to the early 1920s. In 1936, this substance, called collagen hydrolysate, received the GRAS (generally recognized as safe) classification. In recent years, collagen hydrolysate has been on the market in Germany and elsewhere in Europe as a home remedy and a treatment for diseases of the skeletal system and joints.

Only recently available in the United States, this is unlike anything else currently available. A protein derived from bovine collagen, collagen hydrolysate consists of a series of 18 amino acids joined together in chains by peptide bonds. These amino acids are the same ones that make up the framework of human cartilage, contributing to its configuration, flexibility, and strength.

In other words, this substance supplies your cartilage with the nutrients necessary to metabolize (or "use up") old chondrocytes and synthesize new ones. Test after test demonstrates its safety and effectiveness.

Animals fed collagen hydrolysate experienced such significant cartilage growth that researchers could measure it with a ruler! In a controlled study done in 1993 at the Veterinary University in Hanover, Germany, researchers measured a significant increase in thickness in just a few months. Although it's hard to measure cartilage growth in humans, researchers assume the same mechanism is at work as occurs in lab animals.

In one study, 356 people suffering from arthritis in one or more joints — knees, hips, spine — took 1 tablespoon of collagen hydrolysate, mixed with fruit juice, daily. The treatment period lasted from three months to six or even 12 months. Effectiveness was measured on the basis of subjective statements, reduction in the use of NSAIDs, and the abatement in frequency of steroid injections.

Test results: A whopping 99.2 percent of the patients reported "good" or "very good" results. Those with knee pain were completely free of complaints after six months of treatment, without side effects. The researchers concluded that collagen hydrolysate had the strongest pain-relieving effects in those suffering with degeneration of the knee and finger joints.

In another study, 60 patients with youthful chondropathia patellae (a disease of the kneecap cartilage) were treated with collagen hydrolysate for three months. The patients were examined after one, two, and three months. Eighty-six percent reported greater ease in climbing stairs, and 58 percent were free of pain while at rest. At the end of the three months, 75 percent of the patients were free of pain. The researchers concluded that cartilage regeneration occurred in 80 percent of the cases.

Collagen hydrolysate is effective against both rheumatoid arthritis and osteoarthritis

In osteoarthritis, cartilage cells fail to regenerate. Collagen hydrolysate, however, helps to regenerate those tissues by providing the necessary nutrients. Rheumatoid arthritis is an immune-disorder disease. Rather than suppressing the symptoms (which is what steroids do), collagen hydrolysate helps to compensate for destroyed cartilage cells. It fights to outdo the deleterious effects of the disease itself.

If you've just been diagnosed with arthritis of any kind. . .

Collagen hydrolysate can help to halt the wearing down of cartilage, and it may help you prevent further damage. In fact, the earlier you start taking it, the better — especially if you suffer from osteoarthritis, which is degenerative. By nature, a degenerative illness has more potential for cure when caught early on. Even though sufferers of all stages and all forms of arthritis can benefit, collagen hydrolysate is more beneficial and works faster when it is used in the initial stages.

If you've had arthritis for years, consider trying collagen hydrolysate to help slow its progression. It's not too late to help to relieve your suffering. In all the clinical studies, a significant number of sufferers were able to reduce or eliminate their need for conventional painkillers.

If you exercise regularly, even if you only walk a few days a week, collagen hydrolysate may help you minimize the damage to your joints, enabling you to get all the benefits of exercise without risking further damage! If you want to protect your joint health at any age, collagen hydrolysate can serve as a preventive measure to protect and maintain your cartilage.

Actions:
- Contains the amino acids necessary to build new cartilage tissue
- Helps to compensate for cartilage cells destroyed by the immune system

Benefits:
- Helps to relieve severe joint pain
- Improves flexibility
- Reduces the need for prescription and nonprescription medications
- Helps prevent further damage to cartilage tissues

Collagen hydrolysate is a totally new frontier in the treatment of arthritis. A very high percentage of arthritis sufferers who participated in the clinical studies experienced remarkable relief from pain and other symptoms. The recommended dosage is 7 to 10 grams (1 rounded tablespoon) per day, mixed with the beverage of your choice. (It can be bitter! Apple juice helps, as does 1 teaspoon of beet crystals.) For purchasing information, see the "Guide to Sources and Availability," page 167.

Chapter 12

Larreastat: Relief for Victims of Herpes and Rheumatoid Arthritis

In one of the most exciting developments of the decade, researchers recently released their findings on a new, natural product that has been shown to be 99.7 percent effective in the relief of symptoms brought on by the herpes viruses.

If you think that this good news applies only to a few, you may be surprised to learn that, according to recent estimates, up to 90 percent of the population may be infected with one or more of the many herpes viruses. These viruses can lie dormant for years before exhibiting any symptoms, and unsuspecting carriers can easily infect others.

When triggered by stress, infections, or diseases like cancer, herpes viruses can manifest themselves as cold sores, genital lesions, chicken pox, and shingles. Various strains of the virus have also been linked to mononucleosis, chronic fatigue syndrome, and Kaposi's sarcoma, a deadly type of skin cancer frequently, but not exclusively, affecting people with AIDS.

In addition, there is a growing body of evidence that a herpes virus called cytomegalovirus (CMV) plays a causal role in cardiovascular disease. About 75 percent of Americans over 60 carry CMV, with no observable symptoms. But if the virus is "turned on," it appears to play a factor in the clogging of artery walls.[1] Possible triggers include balloon angioplasty and heart-transplant surgery.

And so it was for good reason that researchers in Arizona were elated at the results of studies, confirmed by independent clinical tests, showing that a new "botaniceutical" product derived from the Larrea bush could cripple these insidious viruses without side effects of any kind. By contrast, side effects of acyclovir (Zorivax), the drug commonly prescribed to manage herpes symptoms, include headaches, seizures, coma, nausea, vomiting, and diarrhea. More importantly, prolonged or repeated use of acyclovir can actually encourage the proliferation of drug-resistant strains of the herpes virus.

An ancient desert bush yields this remarkable healing agent

This new preparation is made from an ancient desert bush, Larrea tridentata, used medicinally for centuries by Native Americans as well as early European settlers of the southwestern United States. According to Native American legend, it was the first plant created at the beginning of the world. Scientists have in fact validated that these shrubs are among the oldest living plants on earth, some plants dating back to over 12,000 years ago.

---

[1] Nieto Javier, et. al., "CMV infection as a risk factor for carotid intimal-medial thickening," *Circulation*, vol. 94, no. 5, 1996, pp. 922-7; S.E. Epstein, et. al., "The role of infection in restenosis and atherosclerosis," *Lancet*, vol. 348, Suppl. 1, 1996, pp. 13-17.

Dramatic Relief from Herpes Symptoms

The new Larrea product is formulated both as a topical lotion that can be applied directly to herpes lesions and as a nutritional supplement that can be used to help avert impending outbreaks or to speed healing. Here are only a few of the dozens of successful outcomes confirmed in recent clinical trials:

- A woman suffering from recurrent oral herpes previously used acyclovir with only mixed results. After a single application of the Larrea preparation, lesions were completely healed in 12 hours. Pain and swelling were relieved immediately.
- A 90-year-old woman had Kaposi's sarcoma lesions that covered her body from head to toe. Lesions on her lower extremities were so advanced that one toe had already been amputated. Acyclovir was used without success. After three weeks of treatment twice daily with Larreastat lotion, the lesions on her arm, face, and feet had completely cleared.
- A clinic in Philadelphia treated numerous patients with severe herpes simplex 1 and 2 and zoster (shingles) with both the Larreastat lotion and capsules. They report a 100 percent

success rate, usually within 24-48 hours. The clinicians also reported success using the lotion to avert impending outbreaks, which are usually signaled by a tingling sensation.

- A woman with oral herpes typically had outbreaks lasting three to seven days. When she applied the lotion to a new blister, the pain, swelling, and blistering were gone in one day.
- Shingles sufferers who were treated with Larreastat reported complete relief within minutes.

In dozens of case histories reviewed, one phrase appeared repeatedly: **complete resolution of the episode within 24 hours.** No side effects were reported by any subjects.

Traditionally, Larrea was used to treat infections, snakebites, burns, rheumatism, bronchitis, colds and viruses, and digestive disorders. The phenomenon of an all-purpose natural panacea is not a new one to Health Sciences Institute members. A wide range of effective applications is the hallmark of a natural remedy. These do not work through a single, isolated action, as do our modern pharmaceuticals, but through the varied and synergistic actions of myriad phytochemical compounds.

Clearly, the Larrea shrub, also known in the South-west as the creosote bush and to herbalists as chaparral, is a potent natural healer. Listed in the *Pharmacopoeia of the United States* from 1842 to 1942, chaparral was widely used to treat acne, eczema, venereal and urinary infections, and even certain types of cancer, particularly leukemia.[2] In the 1960s, promising research on the antitumor properties of one of chapparal's chief constituents was abandoned when long-term use in lab animals suggested toxicity.[3] In the early 1990s, a few cases of hepatitis were tied to use of the herb and the FDA requested a voluntary ban on products containing raw chapparal. (Scientists later determined the cases to be unrelated to chapparal use.)[4]

As we have noted before, the fact that something is natural does not mean that it is necessarily harmless. Herbs can be extremely potent, as any student of herbal medicine can attest, and it is possible for an herb to have a toxic effect. Nonetheless, one group of scientists refused to abandon the healing potential of chaparral and continued to search for a way to isolate the beneficial properties of the Larrea bush.

After a decade of research, it appears they have succeeded. Researchers identified a matrix of natural chemicals that appear to be responsible for Larrea's medicinal qualities. Through a proprietary process, they have purified, concentrated, and solubilized these phytochemicals, documented their biological activity, and thoroughly tested them for toxicity of any kind.

---

[2] Andrew Chavallier, *The Encylopedia of Medicinal Plants*, vol. 21, 1997, p. 224.
[3] Varro Tyler, Ph.D., *The Honest Herbal*, 1993, p. 87.
[4] Michael Castleman, "Herbal Healthwatch," *Herb Quarterly*, Spring 1996, p. 6.

The oxidative components of the raw plant believed to be responsible for any toxicity have been eliminated. The result is a natural product that exploits all of the healing potential attributed for centuries to this desert shrub but, according to extensive testing, is safe. Even at doses five times the equivalent human dose, test animals remained in excellent health. Enzyme studies on liver and kidney functions showed no ill effects.

How a herpes treatment can help relieve rheumatoid arthritis

Although the remarkable results of this new product for herpes sufferers are stealing the headlines, there have been equally dramatic reports of relief for rheumatoid arthritis sufferers. An 18-year-old patient suffering from juvenile rheumatoid arthritis for seven years got only minimum relief from even high doses of prescription anti-inflammatories. Upon rising in the morning, the patient was so stiff that he could not walk down the stairs. After using Larreastat capsules for only two weeks, this young man is now playing basketball and holding a full-time summer job.

A 70-year-old California woman with chronic rheumatoid arthritis and long-standing pain and immobility in her knee joint reported over 90 percent relief from pain and swelling and could walk normally again after using Larreastat capsules for two weeks. Numerous other patients of collaborating physicians report dramatic improvements.

How can this preparation be so effective for such

seemingly unrelated conditions as herpes and rheumatoid arthritis? For the same reason that the Larrea plant has been used successfully for centuries for a wide range of conditions. Larrea is rich in a powerful antioxidant lignan called nordihydroguaiaretic acid (NDGA), as well as several other chemically related lignans. Lignans are phytochemicals that show significant antioxidant, anti-inflammatory, antiviral, and antimicrobial properties. In fact, before the modern food industry developed cheaper, synthetic preservatives, NDGA was widely used as a food preservative. It prevents the oxidation of fats and oils in foods, thereby inhibiting the growth of a wide variety of bacteria, yeast, and fungi.

Clearly, Larrea's strong antiviral action makes it a useful weapon against the herpes viruses. But NDGA has also been shown to inhibit 5-lipoxygenase, an enzyme involved in the biochemical process known as the inflammatory cascade. This suggests why Larrea has such a dramatic impact on the symptoms of rheumatoid arthritis, a chronic inflammation caused by the

Actions:
- Inhibits a critical enzyme in the inflammation process
- Prevents oxidative damage
- Strengthens capillaries

Benefits:
- Alleviates pain and inflammation
- Inhibits growth of viruses, bacteria, yeast, and fungi
- Enhances the transport of nutrients

overactivity of the inflammatory cascade in the body.

Furthermore, Larrea is a source of over two dozen flavonoid compounds, many of which are not found in any other known dietary source. These chemicals, which work synergistically with other antioxidant vitamins, especially vitamin C, provide further antioxidant, anti-inflammatory, and antiviral properties. Flavonoids also work to strengthen capillaries, enhancing the transport of nutrients to the tissues of the body.

Because Larreastat products have shown such remarkable ability against diseases for which there are currently so few effective treatments, they represent an important new botanaceutical development. Although preliminary results indicate that this super-purified formula is free of the problems that have been associated with the use of chaparral, the effects of long-term, wide-scale use have yet to be established. For now, a conservative approach dictates use of the preparation on an as-needed basis only, avoiding long-term use until after further studies are concluded. Fortunately, the product is notably fast-acting, making long-term use unnecessary. Currently available through only a limited number of distributors, Larreastat should be available through pharmacies and health-food stores by the end of 1998. See the "Guide to Sources and Availability," page 167.

Chapter 13

Cardiocysteine: Reduce Your Risk of Heart Disease

One in every 2.4 Americans dies from heart disease. To put it plainly, if you don't die from it, someone very close to you will. Even though "only" one in every four Americans today has any of the symptoms — chest pain, high blood pressure, or exertional pain — every man and woman in America has some degree of heart disease. It takes a while to reach deadly levels, but it'll get there.

Whether you know it or not, you may already have heart disease. And you won't find the total protection you need in a garlic or fish-oil capsule. . . any more than you'll find it in a beta-blocker or calcium channel blocker. Neither will you find protection in the ever-popular low-fat diets.

All around the world, crossing genetic and environmental borders, cultures with exceptionally low rates of heart disease have enjoyed and continue to enjoy diets loaded with high-fat, high-cholesterol foods — from the French, with their high-fat cheeses and butter sauces, to the people from northern India, who consume a very high percentage of their calories as butter!

And that's to say nothing of the Myskoke, a group of American Indians, and many other nonindustrialized populations, such as the Eskimos, who consume huge amounts of dietary cholesterol — and have high blood cholesterol — but have very low rates of death from heart disease.

Cholesterol is not the villain

The simple truth is that cholesterol is *not* the deadly threat you may think it is! Aside from the fact that cholesterol is necessary for everything from the production of sex hormones to bile synthesis. . . it simply does not clog up your arteries unless it has something to attach to: a tear, a rough surface, a ridge, a sharp turn.

On that ridge or bump, cholesterol, blood products, and calcium begins to accumulate. These are the blood traps that lead to such problems as impotence, poor memory, heart attack, stroke, and even death.

Harvard's "underground" theory of heart disease

Over 30 years ago, Dr. Kilmer McCully initiated the research that eventually led to the biggest breakthrough in the treatment and prevention of heart disease of our time. McCully, a professor at Harvard Medical College, was researching the causes of arteriosclerosis — then, as now, the No.1 killer of both men and women in America. Dr. McCully suspected that something critical was missing form the mainstream theory on heart disease and, in 1969, proposed the first homocysteine theory of that ailment.

Thirty years and hundreds of studies later, we now know that there is a definite link between homocysteine levels in the blood and heart disease.

Homocysteine can kill—if you don't know how to control it

Your body forms homocysteine when you eat food containing an amino acid called methionine, which is present in all animal and vegetable protein. As part of the digestive process, methionine is broken down into homocysteine. As long as certain helper nutrients are present, homocysteine converts back to methionine, or to another amino acid called cystathionine. (Both are harmless.)

Early research showed that vitamin B-6 is one of the key helper nutrients necessary for normalizing homocysteine levels. When B-6 is low in the blood, homocysteine is high. Unfortunately, the typical American diet is low in vitamin B-6 and high in methionine. And because of food processing, it's virtually impossible to get adequate B-6 in the North American diet.

As McCully discovered early on in his research, homocysteine is even deadlier than had been imagined. It knocks out a mechanism in your artery cells, called "contact inhibition," that keeps the smooth muscle cells just below the inner wall of the artery from growing too rapidly.

At this stage, the smooth muscle cells begin multiplying too fast — just as some forms of cancer do! This creates a bulge that pushes other cells apart and protrudes into the artery, making atherosclerosis possible. The inner wall becomes uneven and rough at this spot, and the buildup of plaque begins.

McCully went even further to suggest that fat in the diet is only a "secondary complication" and that homocysteine overload is the "initial pathogenic factor." Simply put. . . you should be just as concerned— if not more so — over your homocysteine level as you are over your cholesterol level!

Since McCully first proposed his theory on heart disease, the evidence has mounted little by little, showing that. . .

McCully was right all along!

A team of Seattle researchers showed that injections of homocysteine rapidly caused early signs of arteriosclerosis in baboons. The researchers reported that the cells just beneath the artery wall were mutating and reproducing at a wild rate and that this wild growth was destroying the arterial wall! After just one week of high levels of homocysteine in the baboons' blood, 23 percent of their artery walls were lost. The researchers found that the higher the level of homocysteine and the more severely injured the inner artery wall, the more severe the signs of arteriosclerosis. Again: Cholesterol levels were *not* correlated to the destruction of the arteries; cholesterol levels were secondary!

In another study, researchers at the University of Wisconsin's Department of Nutritional Science studied the connection between methionine and B-6 in the diet. For the first 14 days, they gave six male subjects a high-protein diet, supplemented with 2 milligrams of B-6 a day. During that time they found no homocysteine in the urine of the subjects. The researchers then took away the B-6 supplements but kept the high-protein diet the same. By the 21st day, all six men had high levels of homocysteine in their urine. At the end of the 21-day period, the B-6 supplements (2 milligrams per day) were added back into the diet, and the homocysteine levels dropped dramatically in all participants.

It didn't end with B-6. Other researchers uncovered similar links between homocysteine and folic acid, and between homocysteine and B-12, and they found that you need all three nutrients to keep homocysteine levels down.

A study at the Titus County Memorial Hospital, Mount Pleasant, Texas, showed that high homocysteine levels are a risk factor for atherosclerosis and that atherosclerosis is strongly associated with deficiencies of vitamin B-6, folate, and cobalamin (B-12). In that study, the patients who were given vitamin B-6 alone were able to reduce their risk of chest pain and heart attack by 73 percent vs. those who did not add B-6. Those who took B-6 lived an average of eight years longer than those who didn't!

Here's what you need to do TODAY!

You can't ensure healthy, effective levels of B-6, B-12 and folic acid through diet alone. B-6, for example, is destroyed by heating, dehydration, and all other types of food processing. Frighteningly, 80 percent of food consumed by Americans is processed! The average loss of B-6 from freezing fruits and fruit juices is about 15 percent, and from canning, 38 percent. Processed and refined grains lose 51 to 94 percent. Processed meats — which are high in methionine — lose 50 to 75 percent. Food processing causes comparable losses of folic acid and B-12.

Americans are so deficient in these nutrients that even the Food and Drug Administration (FDA) and the Centers for Disease Control (CDC) have stepped in to launch campaigns to get you to increase your intake through supplementation.

Unfortunately, we've discovered that most multivitamin formulas fall short. They simply don't have enough B-6, B-12, or folic acid to be effective in reducing your homocysteine levels.

There is one high-quality supplement, called Cardiocysteine Formula, that is based on the latest homocysteine research. Each tablet provides 800 mcg of folic acid, 500 mcg of B-12 and 25 mcg of B-6. In addition, the formula includes additional nutrients that aid in the metabolism of these crucial heart-protective nutrients. See the "Guide to Sources and Availability" on page 167 for availability.

A final word of caution

We are not saying that homocysteine overload is the only cause of heart disease. There may be other ways in which atherosclerosis is initiated. But all the evidence is there for your scrutiny. You can drastically decrease the likelihood of atherosclerosis by adding to your daily regimen nutrients designed to reverse homocysteine levels in your blood.

Chapter 14

Oxygen Plus: The Healing Power of Oxygen

Various forms of oxygen therapy have been promoted by many alternative medicine practitioners for decades. By increasing the amount of oxygen in your system, you can empower your immune system and provide life and energy to every cell. It has been widely accepted that oxygen deficiency is the greatest cause of disease. Yet antioxidants, including many vitamins that have a primarily antioxidant function, have long been recognized as offering a wide range of health benefits. The two theories seem to work to opposite ends. Which do we want, oxidation or antioxidation? And can they work together?

The answer is very simple. In the body, oxygen can be present in two different forms with two very different effects. Positively charged "free" oxygen molecules are very destructive to most of the chemicals in the body. These so-called "free radicals" are the ones we attempt to neutralize with dietary and supplemental antioxidants. A wide range of diseases, especially chronic degenerative conditions related to aging, are now thought to be linked to failures of the antioxidant systems that protect the integrity of our DNA against oxidative damage.

The Many Uses of Oxygen Plus

Water Treatment: For safe drinking water, use 5 to 20 drops per 8-ounce glass: 5 drops for Baby, 20 for Dad. For water storage, use 8 to 12 drops per gallon. Milk and juices: 10 to 15 drops per quart will extend freshness up to several weeks in most cases.

Skin Cuts and Small Burns: Superficial cuts and small area burns may be treated one time only with a few drops placed directly on the wound to help stop bleeding and/or reduce pain. This will also reduce the risk of infection. Do not use directly on sunburns without diluting: one part liquid oxygen to 20 parts pure water.

Fever Blisters, Cold Sores, Herpes: Use 1 to several drops dabbed directly on the wound, one time only, twice weekly.

Mouth and Teeth: Place 5 or 6 drops on your toothbrush while brushing your teeth. Use 5 drops in a half-ounce of water for a disinfecting mouthwash, swishing between your teeth.

Infections, Flu, Viruses: At the first sign of illness, melt 1 teaspoon of honey in 1 ounce of hot water. Add 50 drops of liquid oxygen and drink. Repeat three times daily the first day. On the second and third days, repeat, but reduce drops to 25 each time. In addition, drink 3 glasses of water daily, each containing 20 drops. For a person weighing only 70 to 100 pounds, cut the dose in half.

> **Warning:** Don't put this directly into your eye or ear. If you do want to work on an infection in one of those sensitive areas, please dilute the product. Aloe vera juice is an excellent medium for this purpose. (A solution of 1 drop of oxygen to 5 drops of aloe usually works.)

But the other side of the coin is that insufficient oxygen is often blamed for these same degenerative diseases! In this case, however, we are referring to a lack of negatively charged oxygen molecules, which oxygenate and enrich the blood and tissues of the body, enhancing nutrient uptake and stimulating the body's immune-system functions.

Oxygen Plus is a chemical oxygen supplier that contains negatively charged oxygen molecules, actually increasing the amount of available oxygen to the body without supplying dangerous free-radical oxygen.

Chemical oxygen suppliers are effective antibacterial agents. Oxygen was deadly to anaerobic bacteria billions of years ago, and it remains so today. Chemical sources of oxygen also have a desirable effect in altering the body's pH toward the basic side, away from the acidic. Wheat products, coffee, soda, and meat all contribute to a diet that is far too acidic for optimal health.

However, the remarkable effects of Oxygen Plus on conditions like diabetes, emphysema, and

Alzheimer's disease are most likely due to its ability to supply additional oxygen energy for a wide range of cellular functions.

Oxygen enhancer produces surprising results for emphysema, diabetes, and more

People with emphysema, for example, report dramatic improvement from using Oxygen Plus. (The working protocol for emphysema appears to be 20 drops of Oxygen Plus, three times a day, with juice — to facilitate entry into the lungs. The quantity can be decreased after success is achieved.)

Diabetic Keith Whitmore, from Sandy, Utah, found that his blood-sugar levels dropped and then stabilized forevermore with the use of this oxygen supplement. Michael Purles of Salt Lake City noted that he eliminated the visual problems that had been plaguing him for years. His wife Gerry got rid of her sinus infections. Cliff Foley of Ridgefield, Washington, reported that his congestive heart failure took a complete turnabout. The list goes on.

Remember that the power of oxygen is its ability to help stop the progression of toxins, viruses, and bacteria, whether inside your body or out. There are many other uses of oxygen as an external detoxifier:

- If you are stung by any kind of insect, or are bitten by any kind of animal that may have venom, dropping some of this liquid onto the bite or sting will neutralize the poisons almost immediately.

- You can also try this solution on rashes caused by stinging nettle, poison oak, or poison ivy. These toxins draw on your own oxygen supply because of the free radicals set in motion.
- When oxygen is applied directly to a bruise and massaged in, the toxins in the lymphatic system, blood, and the skin area are neutralized. This helps a bruise heal faster and gets rid of some of the pain.

Keep in mind that oxygen alone cannot cure any condition. Its true power is in enhancing your body's ability to function efficiently, absorb and utilize important nutrients, and eliminate toxins. Used in combination with powerful immune-system stimulants like lactoferrin (see Chapter 1) and medicinal mushrooms (see Chapter 3), Oxygen Plus helps build a formidable defense against today's toxic environment and our overburdened immune systems. Needless to say, when working to resolve a serious health problem, you should consult a qualified health practitioner familiar with the specifics of your situation.

Please turn to the "Guide to Sources and Availability" on page 167 for information on obtaining liquid oxygen.

Chapter 15

DHA: Boost Your Brain Power

One of today's most popular heart supplements, the omega-3 fish oil docosahexaenoic acid (DHA, not to be confused with the hormone DHEA) is likely to be tomorrow's most sought-after brain pill. In Norway, doctors regularly prescribe DHA to lower cholesterol. In the United States, it's available in health-food stores and is known for its ability to greatly lower the risk of a sudden deadly heart attack. It's also well-known as an important nutrient for pregnant women, since DHA is crucial to fetal brain development.

The latest research from Japan demonstrates why DHA is also necessary to maintain optimum brain functioning in adults, and why it could turn out to be critical for the prevention and possible reversal of Alzheimer's disease!

Keeping your brain alive, active, and alert — cell by cell

You have approximately 14 billion brain cells, each of which connects and "talks" to other brain cells by sending signals through electrical "arms" called synapses. This communication is the basis for learning and memory, as well as for sending messages of pain and pleasure throughout your body. When the arms between brain cells are flexible and pliant, the communication operates at its best. Studies show that DHA is critical to maintaining soft and flexible synapses, thus keeping your brain healthy and active.

When the level of DHA drops, reducing synapse flexibility, the arms become hardened and signals are transmitted more slowly. Researchers in Japan have recently observed that the absence of DHA is associated with many cognitive and mental-health conditions, such as depression, schizophrenia, and dementia of the Alzheimer's type.

DHA as a treatment for Alzheimer's

Early tests on treatment with DHA have been very promising. In a study performed at Gunma National University in Japan, patients suffering from symptoms of Alzheimer's disease showed a 65 percent improvement in symptoms of dementia with the use of DHA.

In another study, researchers formulated their own omega-3 oil product to make sure it had a very high concentration of DHA (53 percent), because, they write, most of the current "omega-3 fish-oil products are low in DHA content (12 percent) and are primarily marketed for heart disease." The researchers wanted to test the maximum effects of DHA on brain function, so they significantly increased the percentage of DHA and conducted a memory study with lab animals. The results of their 20-day investigation showed that (1) DHA improves memory and (2) the higher the dose, the better the results.

How to choose the best source of DHA

You have to be very particular when you're looking for your DHA supplement, because, as noted, the majority of the fish oils you'll find in the health-food stores have been prepared as heart-health supplements and are *not* going to give your brain the support it needs.

Look for a fish-oil supplement with a high ratio of DHA to EPA. (EPA, eicosapentaoic acid, as you may already know, lowers cholesterol, but it also has an anticlotting effect you want to avoid.) Try to find a supplement derived from tuna; of all the cold-water fish, tuna has the highest DHA content. A good ratio of DHA to EPA would be 25 to 30 percent DHA to 7 percent or less EPA.

Actions:
- Nourishes and supports neural synapses
- Enhances synapse flexibility
- Promotes nerve-signal transmission
- Lowers cholesterol

Benefits:
- Improves memory and mental functioning
- May protect against depression, schizophrenia, and dementia (Alzheimer's disease)
- Reduces the risk of a sudden deadly heart attack

While your body can synthesize most fats, there are a few that are considered "essential" because you must obtain them from food or supplements. DHA is an essential fatty acid. You need to continually refresh your brain's supply. And here's an extra tip for improving your brain health: One study showed that DHA was even more effective for those who eat fish at least five times a week in addition to taking the DHA.

The recommended amount for DHA supplementation is 750 milligrams a day. For purchasing information, see the "Guide to Sources and Availability," page 167.

Chapter 16

ProzaPlex: Nature's Alternative to Prozac

In one of the most widely publicized break-throughs of the decade, St. John's wort (or Hypericum perforatum) has staged a coup in Europe, virtually replacing chemical antidepression drugs as the treatment of choice for depression. "The herbal antidepressants have literally taken over the Prozac marketplace in Germany," writes Dr. Daniel Beilin, an herbalist and acupuncturist in Aptos, California.

There is now little doubt concerning the effectiveness of St. John's wort. An article in *Clinical Research* (vol. 313, no. 7052, pp. 253-8) reported results from 23 randomized trials involving a total of 1,757 subjects with mild to moderately severe depressive disorders. Fifteen of these studies were placebo-controlled, and eight compared Hypericum with another drug treatment. Hypericum extracts outperformed the placebo by a factor of 2.7 and were at least as effective as standard antidepressant preparations.

A double-blind, placebo-controlled study, representative of several published in Germany, found a 70 percent response rate among 97 outpatients who received 100 to 120 milligrams of Hypericum extract. "Treatment resulted in an appreciable improvement in the symptoms of depression, and the 70 percent response rate corresponded to that of chemical antidepressants. The substance was extremely well tolerated, and no side effects were reported by any of the patients" (*Fortschritte der Medizin*, vol. 113, no. 28, pp. 404-8).

And from another article in *Fortschritte der Medizin* (vol. 113, no. 25, pp. 354-5): "Recent studies have shown that [St. John's wort] is clinically effective for the treatment of the symptoms of depression. It has proved superior to placebos and equally as beneficial as stan-

---

New St. John's wort formula adds important botanicals

- Kava kava is a Polynesian drink with psychoactive properties, used extensively for medicinal purposes in some traditional island cultures. It appears to be nonaddictive with few known side effects and may act like tricyclic drugs, although the mechanism is not known.
- Schizandra is believed to protect the liver against oxidative damage and improve its capacity to safeguard against foreign enzymes introduced by treatment.
- Zinc salts help control the permeability of the "blood-brain barrier" and are believed to improve the effectiveness of Hypericum.
- Orchid root is another psychoactive herb found to be useful in rehabilitation—from addiction to other stimulant drugs.

dard medication, over which it has a clear advantage in terms of side effects. It follows that, on the basis of our present knowledge, St. John's wort can be recommended for use as an antidepressant."

A good thing made even better

Although it has been St. John's wort that has received most of the attention in the mainstream press, there is, in fact, a large class of natural, traditional, and mostly underutilized herbal treatments that have very definite psychoactive properties.

Taking the St. John's wort revolution one step farther, the Health Sciences Institute has found and evaluated a unique formula called ProzaPlex that combines Hypericum with several other very important herbs. The results of human trials indicate that the ingredients in this little-known formula seem to be even more effective than Hypericum alone.

In addition to Hypericum perforatum, ProzaPlex contains kava kava root (Piper methysticum), Schizandra chinensis, passionflower (Passiflora incarnata), zinc salts, and orchid root extract (Cypripedium).

Caution: Because of Hypericum's suppression of response to light, there is increased danger of serious sunburn while using it. Keep this in mind, especially if you are using any photosensitizing drugs. Also, the mechanism that increases dopamine levels inhibits prolactin, so nursing mothers should avoid Hypericum.

The multiplicity of modes of action sheds light on the real differences between drug and herbal treatment: The drug manufacturer attempts to isolate a single action and to refine and purify a single chemical product that will affect that action and do a minimum of other things. Prozac is a good example. Earlier antidepressants inhibited the reduction of both serotonin and norepinephrine. But the second mode of action caused side effects like drowsiness, dry mouth, and blurred vision. So that part was eliminated, and Prozac probably works through one mechanism alone.

An herbal treatment based on Hypericum along with other synergistic herbs, on the other hand, spreads the effect over a much greater number of elements in the total neurological and hormonal picture, making it far less likely that any one resulting action will produce unintended and undesirable side effects. The herbal treatment combines Hypericum with other herbs that have overlapping modes of action. That way, the probability of developing a tolerance for one substance, leading to diminishing results, is greatly reduced.

Here's a sampling of the reports we've received from those who have tried ProzaPlex:

"After two weeks on Prozaplex, my mood totally changed. Little things that used to irritate me don't anymore. I have a brighter outlook on life, despite a big emotional upset that happened." E.J.

"When I was on Zoloft, I felt groggy. It felt like a wet blanket over me. Now, with ProzaPlex, I am able to think more clearly, and function much better." J.S.

"I have been severely depressed for 20 years. I started using ProzaPlex three weeks ago and within 72 hours I felt as though I could see a window of light — a pathway of a new stability and increased control of my sadness." D.P.

"I have been on other St. John's products for a year or so. I decided now that I am stable I would try ProzaPlex. With ProzaPlex, I feel as if I have gotten to the 'next level' of the feeling of wellness. Whatever is added, maybe it's the Orchid extract, I feel more capable in my life as well as even brighter." D.S.

See page 167 for the "Guide to Sources and Availability" for this new formula and other St. John's Wort products.

Chapter 17

The Plant-Based Nutrition System: More Than a Weight-Loss Aid

This may be the only tool you'll ever need to switch on your fat-burning metabolism, switch off your nagging cravings, and lose weight for a lifetime. It's a new food-concentrate program that nourishes your body with a wholeness no diet or supplement program can match. By adding this weight-loss formula to your daily regimen, you'll satisfy your body's nutritional needs with minimal calories: your cravings will vanish, and you just may slip naturally into fat-burning mode. Side benefits of this program include better digestion, normal blood-sugar levels, daily detoxification, and enhanced resistance to disease.

This is not just a weight-loss aid. It's a daily nutrition survival kit. It can, and should, be used by everyone. But a major added benefit of this program is that, if you need to, it will help you lose weight—for good!

The Plant-based Nutrition System satisfies your body's requirements for every basic nutritional demand, by using nature's most nutritionally abundant and biochemically active plant foods, grown in season.

Wherever possible, they are also organic, nonhybrid, and not crossbred.

The Plant-based Nutrition System consists of four products derived from whole foods:

- a primary source for proteins, fiber, and essential fatty acids, called Pro Fiber EFA
- a dehydrated fruit drink, called Bio Fruit
- a dehydrated yellow vegetable drink, called Phyto Carrot
- a dehydrated deep-green leafy-vegetable drink, called Best of Greens

This is not just dehydrated space food. The nuts, seeds, and grains in the Pro Fiber EFA supplement are simply ground up. The fruit and vegetable mixes are not isolates but whole foods that have been vacuum-extracted. These procedures separate these products from so many others in the marketplace.

The benefits of dried whole foods

When the dehydrating temperature is low, drying retains more nutritional value than toasting, roasting, steaming, baking, or frying. Since most of the water content is removed in the drying process, you're left with a food that has a significantly increased density of many nutrients on a portion-for-portion basis. This is particularly true of the more stable nutrients, such as minerals.

If you had to, you could live on this product alone!

Of course, the total plan falls short of the number of calories needed. (As you'll see in a moment, the fact that it is low in calories, yet packed with nutrients, is one of the reasons it helps you lose weight and keep it off.)

Take a closer look at the nutrients you get:

Fats and Oils

Instead of fats from sweets (as our infamous Food Pyramid allows), you'll get omega-3, -6, and -9 oils in the form of flax, chia, pumpkin, hemp, quinoa, sprouted grains, and spirulina —all present in the Pro Fiber EFA.

The chia seed, under cultivation in Mexico and in the southwestern United States for centuries, has phenomenal protein and oil qualities. Chia contains a natural antioxidant that helps to prevent the oil from becoming rancid. The pumpkin seed has an ingredient that helps to shrink the male prostate. Hemp seed has high amounts of essential fatty acids (EFAs). All of these seeds are very important for heart tissue. They lower high cholesterol and strengthen connective tissue, thereby reducing heart-attack risk.

These fats are also crucial to losing weight without having to struggle with cravings or hunger pangs.

Protein

Unlike the Food Pyramid, which encourages a variety of dairy products, meats, nuts, and beans as protein sources, the Pro Fiber EFA is all-vegetarian, so it's free of processed animal fat. The protein sources — flax, chia, pumpkin, quinoa, spirulina, fennel, rice bran, and sprouted grains — are all lightweight, enzyme-containing proteins. Together, they supply the eight essential amino acids, a rare find in vegetarian foods.

Incidentally, you may notice that some of the foods in the protein category are also listed in the fat group. And you'll see them again in the fiber listing. These super foods naturally provide well-balanced nourishment, covering many bases!

Fruits

Most people eat apples, bananas, and oranges and think they're getting the fruit nutrients they need. But these are not the fruits that have the most powerful impact. The Bio Fruit drink contains extracts from:

- elderberries, with immune-boosting phyto-chemicals called polyphenols
- pomegranates, with phytoestrogens promoting hormone balance
- citrus peels, the richest source of bioflavonoids, which build collagen and assist in vitamin C absorption and utilization
- grape seeds, known for the powerful anti-oxidant pycnogenol
- bilberries, with anthocyanisides, phyto-chemicals that improve eyesight
- palmetto berries, with lipids and active sterols known to shrink an enlarged prostate (You also get the prostate-health benefits of the pumpkin seed in the Pro Fiber EFA. The developer of the system found that the palmetto berries and the pumpkin

seeds don't combine well in one product but work better in their own natural categories.)

- cranberries, with polycyanadines, well-known for preventing and treating urinary-tract infections
- apples, with soluble fiber to help remove waste

The fruit drink is low in sugar, so it can be used to supply these health-promoting fruit phytochemicals for diabetics, hypoglycemics, or anyone else on a fruit-restricted diet.

Vegetables

This program gives you the benefits of deep-green leafy vegetables as well as yellow varieties. With the Best of Greens drink, you automatically meet your requirement for phytochemically active greens — a goal advocated by our government and our medical community, but rarely met. Among the greens are kale, wheatgrass, spirulina, sea vegetables, barley, and dandelion greens. This mix serves up natural sources of calcium, trace minerals, chlorophyll, enzymes, and other phytochemicals — so you're getting nature's most powerful antidotes and preventives for cancer, osteoporosis, anemia, and heavy-metal toxicity. It also contains friendly bacteria, including acidophilus, bifidus, and facelum.

The Phyto Carrot drink combines soybean lecithin and soybean sprouts with the most nutritious of the yellow vegetables — carrots, sweet potatoes, and wild yams — to give you carotenoids, phytoestrogens, and phospholipids.

Breads, Cereals, and Rice

The Pro Fiber EFA also offers the nutritional benefits of seven sprouted grains plus rice bran. The sprouted grains are grown in season, not in a hot house. Their enzymes are activated, their proteins convert to free amino acids, their starches change to simple plant sugars, their minerals combine to augment assimilation, their vitamin content increases many times over, and their chlorophyll and carotene content are boosted dramatically.

Rice bran contains a substance called oryzanol, which enables certain cholesterol-controlling enzymes in your liver to function more effectively. LDL-cholesterol levels of test animals maintained on rice-bran oil are significantly lower, while their HDL-cholesterol levels are higher. But the protective properties of oryzanol go beyond that of lowering cholesterol. Oryzanol also reduces deposits of various other unwanted collections in your arteries.

Fiber

The Plant-based Nutrition System gives you a gentle combination of soluble and insoluble fiber from nuts, fruits, beans, grains, seeds, and vegetables. Soluble fiber helps to reduce your LDL cholesterol. Insoluble fiber, the brushes and brooms of the bowel, cleanses and detoxifies your system.

Since you'll get most of your fiber from grains that are high in protein and good-guy fats, and since these grains have their enzymes intact, you're not likely to suffer from the digestive disorders that typically accompany increased fiber intake.

The program also includes a special herbal supplement that acts as an immune booster. It includes garlic, Ginkgo biloba, selenium, and potent antioxidants in a base of dehydrated beet juice.

Here's how the Plant-based Nutrition System helps you lose weight

Conventional weight-loss plans typically rely on diets that cut calories and/or fat — regimens that restrict or eliminate certain foods. Or they may be herbal or prescription medicines that suppress your appetite. These "diets of subtraction" inevitably starve your body calorically and nutritionally. As a result, your genetically programmed anti-starvation mechanism sets in, causing you to burn fuel more slowly and to store more fat. To make matters worse, this is precisely when your cravings surface.

The irresistible urge starts at the cellular level

Your cells, which aren't getting the fat, protein, vitamins, or minerals they need, send an urgent STARVATION message to your brain This powerful message usually leads to images of cake, ice cream, fried chicken, or any high-fat, high-calorie food that generally offers you very little nutritional value! Your good intentions and defenses break down with ease!

Says Health Sciences Institute panel member Dr. Richard Kunin, "A diet that does not supply sufficient fatty acids leads to cravings that most people (rightly) will not ignore. It almost guarantees failure."

As we all know, diets of "subtraction" add pounds in the long run, but the Plant-based Nutrition System is a diet of addition. It provides a high concentration of nutrients with a low concentration of calories, leading to a state of "cellular satisfaction."

In short, you get more energy. . . more muscle. . . normalized blood-sugar levels. . . improved resistance to disease. . . detoxified blood. . . and weight loss without hunger pangs or fatigue.

The program is available in one-, three-, and six-month supplies, at a cost of about $2.60 a day. All three packages include a free, personal-sized battery-run mixer and an instructional manual, including directions on using the system for weight loss, maintenance, and/or fasting and detoxification. See the "Guide to Sources and Availability" on page 167.

Chapter 18

Cig-No: Quit Smoking for the Last Time

"It's easy to quit smoking," goes the old saw. "I've done it many times." This is too tragic to be funny. You're no doubt fully aware of the devastating health effects of smoking. Most smokers who know even a small fraction of the truth about smoking and health want desperately to quit. But nicotine is one of the most addictive drugs on the planet. Smokers can try to compensate for their habit with a healthy lifestyle, optimum nutrition, and intelligent use of supplements, but these measures can never really equal the benefits of quitting.

The Health Sciences Institute has reviewed several products designed to help smokers kick the habit and has come across one homeopathic formula that can actually reduce cravings for cigarettes.

The Cig-No smoking-deterrent system includes a spray, liquid drops, and capsules. All three use the herb Plantago major, which has a long history of medicinal use. Most importantly, Plantago major can create an aversion reaction to tobacco, as documented by several authoritative sources.

The liquid and spray forms of Cig-No, homeopathic preparations administered sublingually (under the tongue), are said to instantly suppress the craving for tobacco. The capsules typically require 20 minutes to act. All three delivery systems can be used interchangeably or as complements to one another.

There is supporting clinical data for the efficacy of Plantago major. A one-day trial conducted in 1992 involving 24 heavy smokers documented an aversion to smoking after participants received a 20 percent tincture of Plantago major at two- or four-hour intervals. The effect was dose-dependent — the more the subjects received, the stronger the aversion. This effect might indeed be enough to increase the success rate for permanent smoking cessation.

This is certainly not the first quitting aid to claim to dislodge the physiological cause of addiction or to create an aversion to tobacco smoke. Yet anecdotal reports passing through our offices suggest that this system actually works better than previous formulations. It definitely offers a nontoxic alternative to the increasingly popular nicotine patches and gums. Turn to the "Guide to Sources and Availability" on page 167.

Chapter 19

Kava Kava: The Feel-Good Herb of the South Pacific

Though kava kava has been around for thousands of years and is widely used as a pharmaceutical in Europe, few in America are keyed in to what this herb can do.

Kava kava (Piper methysticum) is a member of the pepper family. This lush, green plant with heart-shaped leaves grows as high as 8 feet tall before being harvested by the South Pacific islanders.

Islanders drink the pungent juice of the root instead of alcohol at bars. They take kava kava breaks instead of coffee breaks. They drink kava kava juice to celebrate wedding ceremonies. Feuding families drink it to remain calm, helping to resolve their problems. The elderly drink the juice to enhance mental clarity and to relax their muscles. And legend has it that a half coconut shell full of strong kava kava may put you into a deep, dreamless sleep for two hours.

If you have trouble falling asleep, if you wake up in the middle of the night and can't get back to sleep, or if you sleep fitfully all night and rise in the morning feeling exhausted. . . kava kava may be the answer to your prayers.

A potent treatment for serious and disruptive anxiety-related disorders

Make no mistake, this natural intoxicant is also a serious — but safe — herbal medicine. It is used to treat...

- depression
- anxiety and panic attacks
- insomnia
- mood swings

As a natural relaxant that reduces stress, kava kava is also helpful for high blood pressure. And, because it has been shown to have analgesic properties, it may help to relieve any painful condition — headaches, toothaches, and general muscle pain.

A proven folk medicine — backed up by 150 years of research

Proof of kava kava's effectiveness and safety is supported by hundreds (if not thousands) of years of use by the island communities of the South Pacific — from Hawaii to New Zealand. In addition, Western scientific studies on kava kava date as far back as the mid 1800s, when European scientists first began to identify, isolate, and test what they discovered to be the active ingredients: kavalactones.

Although the kava kava plant contains at least 15 different kavalactones, 150 years of research has shown that only six are biochemically active: yangonin, methysticin, kavain, dihydromethysticin (DHM), dihydrokava kavain, and demethosy-yangonin.

It is through these lipid-like substances that kava

kava works its gentle magic.

A potent alternative to prescription sleep aids and antidepressants

As is evident from the popularity of Prozac (the first-ever $2 billion-dollar antidepressant) and the growing class of antianxiety drugs known as benzodiazepines (such as Valium, Halcion, Xanax, and Serax), Americans are in need of a safe, natural mood-relaxing substance.

As many as 22.2 percent of women and 16.9 percent of men in the United States suffer from anxiety disorders, according to the National Foundation for Brain Research.

During any six-month period, 9 million Americans suffer from a depressive illness, says the National Institutes of Mental Health.

It is estimated that 60 percent of American adults experience some degree of sleeplessness as a result of either depression or anxiety. Benzodiazepines, the most commonly prescribed antianxiety drugs, can cause headaches, drowsiness, dizziness, and vertigo and are physically habit-forming. In addition, their effects often diminish over time, making it necessary to increase the dosage.

Kava kava, on the other hand, is nonaddictive and nontoxic when taken at the recommended dosage.

Research has proven that kava kava works — and that it's safe

A number of studies have shown that kava kava relaxes the limbic system, the emotional center of the brain. Like the benzodiazepines, kavalactones act on the small, chickpea-sized organ called the amygdala, which regulates feelings of fear and anxiety and processes memories en route to the cerebral cortex.

Researchers have yet to explain, however, how kava kava produces its relaxing and uplifting response without the side effects and hazards of prescription anti-anxiety drugs. But they do know this:

- **Kava kava is as strong as prescription anti-anxiety drugs, but with NO side effects.** In 1990, a team of German researchers conducted a four-week study that compared the effects of kava kava and oxazapam (a popular benzodiazepine) on 38 patients suffering from anxiety. The kava kava extract reduced symptoms of anxiety as effectively as oxazapam — but with no side effects.

- **Kava kava does *not* inhibit mental function.** In 1993, researchers made use of standardized tests for mental function and reaction time to compare kava kava with benzodiazepine. The study demonstrated that while the benzodiazepine decreased both the quality and the speed of responses to test questions, the kava kava reduced anxiety without interfering with mental clarity. In fact, those who took the kava kava had slightly improved reaction time and recognition.

- **Kava kava outperforms placebos.** In a 1991 study of 58 patients with anxiety, researchers gave half the patients 100 milligrams of a 70 percent kavalactone extract three times a day for four weeks. The other half (the control group) received placebos. Those who took the kava kava extract enjoyed significant relief from their symptoms in just one week. (No side effects were reported.)
- **Kava kava is an effective painkiller.** While it was already well-known that chewing fresh kava kava produced local anesthesia in the chewer's mouth, a team of scientists from the Freiburg University Institute of Pharmacology in Germany, led by J. Meyer, established that one kavalactone in particular, kavain, functions as a superficial anesthetic, as effective as cocaine but completely nontoxic to the tissues.

Kava kava has also proven to help reduce symptoms of depression and anxiety in menopausal women.

Take a lesson — and a cure — from the ancient wisdom of the South Pacific

You can mix kava kava tinctures with herbal tea, take the extract as a capsule or tablet, or take the liquid form under your tongue. (The liquid form works faster, but it may not last as long.) To make sure you're getting an effective dose and product, look for a standardized kava kava extract containing at least 25 to 30 percent kavalactones.

It's *not* dangerous to take an unstandardized supplement, but you won't be able to determine the exact potency and may have to take more of the product to get the desired results.

Though kava kava is readily available in health-food stores, biochemist Herman Lam recently introduced a high-potency extract to the American Academy of Environmental Medicine:

> I studied a number of different kava kava products, but none was as potent as I'd read it should be. When I finally found a product that worked — the Guaranteed Potency Extract — I introduced it at a medical meeting of the American Academy of Environmental Medicine in Boston. We didn't have the capsule form yet, so I offered samples of the liquid variety. Five or six doctors expressed interest in the product, but they were also concerned — they didn't want to fall asleep. I promised it wouldn't put them to sleep, filled their glasses. . . and a few minutes later, one doctor sang out that her headache was gone. Another said that his back pain disappeared. It went on and on. . . the crowd got larger and larger. . .

Recommended amount of kava kava

Though native islanders drink it by the coconut shell, Western science has provided a dosage range for the uninitiated — between 70 and 250 milligrams of kavalactones. Try 70 milligrams for a mild relaxing effect; increase the dosage to 150-250 as a sleep aid.

In terms of standardized supplements, if the preparation you buy contains, for example, 150 mg of standardized kava kava root extract, at 30 percent kavalactones, you're getting 50 mg of kavalactones.

Actions:

- Relaxes the limbic system, the emotional center of the brain
- Act as a natural analgesic

Benefits:

- Reduces stress
- Relieves pain
- Calms anxiety and panic attacks
- Prevents insomnia

A word of caution: Overindulgence in kava kava (310 to 440 grams per week) may lead to liver damage, dry scaly skin, and alterations in red and white blood cells and platelets. (A 1988 study in Australia showed that heavy kava kava drinkers suffered from malnutrition because the kava kava consumption replaced much of the subjects' food intake.)

For information on the availability of kava kava, see the "Guide to Sources and Availability" on page 167.

Section IV

Technology for Health

*A*lthough nature is a great and limitless source of healing substances, sometimes the most exciting breakthroughs in modern, alternative medicine are made in highly sophisticated laboratories, as scientists use the newest technology to examine the complex hormonal, neural, and immunological systems that govern our health.

The blending of science and technology with the holistic and noninvasive principles of natural healing has yielded several high-tech tools that can enhance our health and extend our lives. Learn how to put the best of alternative–medicine technology to work for you.

Chapter 20

Magnetic Field Therapy: The Healing Force Field

The healing tool of the future injects no chemicals into your body, involves neither knife nor plaster cast, and works fast. It relieves pain, floods the inflamed or injured area with nutrients and oxygen-rich blood, enables your body to remove toxins more efficiently, and accelerates your body's natural recovery process.

The healing tool of the future is none other than the magnet. Already used widely in Europe and Asia, magnet therapy is reportedly able to boost your melatonin levels, cure depression, replenish your oxygen-starved heart or gangrenous limb, instantly kill headaches and back pain, and even kill bacteria.

While some of these claims are not yet supported by methodical research, a number of controlled double-blind studies and clinical reports show that magnets (also called "biomagnets") do initiate healing and provide quick pain relief for a number of conditions, namely lower-back pain, shoulder and neck pain, tendonitis, bursitis, headaches, and bone fractures. In some cases, magnet therapy doubles the healing rate.

Charles W. Kennedy Jr., M.D., former president of the Texas Orthopedic Association and current president of MAGNAflex Inc., uses biomagnets to treat patients suffering from lower back pain, tendonitis, bursitis, myofascial pain syndrome, and inflammatory conditions of the hips and legs. Due to the "cost effectiveness" and therapeutic success of magnet therapy, Dr. Kennedy receives 80 to 90 percent reimbursement through insurance providers.

Dr. Kennedy first learned of biomagnets in 1990 when his wife, suffering from severe tennis elbow, was not improving, despite a combination of physical therapy, anti-inflammatory injections, and exercise.

"A mutual friend was at that time promoting the use of biomagnets manufactured in Germany," says Dr. Kennedy. "We bought the device from him, and to my surprise, within two weeks, my wife's tennis-elbow problem was cured. This product has allowed her to resume her active life free of pain and complications related to her injury. When she does get an occasional flare-up of the problem, she reapplies a biomagnet overnight and is able to resume uninhibited activities the following day."

How do magnets work?

You may already be aware that your blood, bones, and organs are brimming with dynamic, charged particles — and biomagnets are not the first health tools to exploit the human-energy field. If you undergo an MRI (magnetic resonance imaging) exam, for example, the hydrogen atoms in your body are temporarily altered by magnetic coils and scanned for signs of abnormality, such as a tumor or cyst.

But for thousands around the world, magnet therapy is being used in many other "unconventional" ways. By mobilizing the body's stores of oxygen, nutrients, and immune chemicals, magnets accelerate the healing of a seemingly unlimited array of illnesses and conditions.

"The blood is chock-full of electrically charged particles," says Dr. Ted J. Zablotsky, president of BIOflex Inc., in Avon, Connecticut. "The reactions to the magnet cause the blood vessel to widen, and more blood comes to the area. It's not a miracle; it just acts like one . . .The principle of physics that all this is based upon is called the Hall effect, which says that if I have a moving electrical current and I put a magnet at right angles with respect to that current, the particles in that current are going to react in a certain predictable way . . .If you have an over-use injury, say tennis elbow, and you increase blood flow to that inflamed area, you're going to relieve the tennis elbow — in less than 12 hours there can be a significant reduction in pain . . .Basically, the magnets cause an increase in blood flow . . .an acceleration of the natural healing process."

In 1991, Dr. Thomas Laser, head physician of the orthopedic department at the Klinic Bavaria in Germany, conducted an extensive double-blind study on the use of magnets on patients with chronic pain (low-back, neck, and shoulder pain). The yearlong study, in which patients were given either magnetized or demagnetized foils, revealed that the effectiveness of the magnetized foils was "unmistakably higher than the placebo effect of the nonmagetized foils applied to the control group."

Seventy percent of those who used the magnetized foils enjoyed pain relief, compared with only 26 percent of those using nonmagnetized foils; 46 percent of those using the magnetized foils were able to reduce their painkillers, compared with only 10 percent in the control group.

In another double-blind study, this one at Barry University in Miami, Florida, in 1993, researchers compared the use of magnetized pads with that of demagnetized pads on patients with heel pain syndrome. Almost 60 percent of those using the magnetized pads enjoyed notable pain relief, vs. just 16 percent of those using the demagnetized pads. Seventy-seven percent of those using the magnetized pads showed improvement in walking, compared with only 16 percent of those using demagnetized pads.

Other conditions for which magnet therapy is reportedly useful include depression, anxiety, phobias, diabetic neuropathy, angina, sinus pain, and insomnia.

Are there risks?

Some physicians believe that the static magnetic field of a biomagnet does little more than block pain signals to the brain. Others have suggested that prolonged exposure could disturb your natural "rhythms," right down to your chromosomes, and that magnets may even cause cancer. In 1987, however, a World

Health Organization study examining over 40 years of research concluded that the type of magnetic field present in a biomagnet does not cause cancer. In terms of strength and exposure time, it is best to follow the manufacturer's recommendations, but be aware that the U.S. Department of Energy recommends that when using a magnet of over 5,000 gauss (a gauss is a unit of measurement for magnetic intensity) you should limit your exposure time to 10 minutes per session.

Therapeutic biomagnets can be as strong as 12,500 gauss and are available in patches, cards, blankets, mattress overlays, insoles, lumbar support belts, and face masks. For more information, contact the Bio-Electromagnetics Institute; 2490 W. Moana Lane; Reno, Nevada 89509-3936; tel. (702) 827-9099. This private nonprofit organization was established to provide research, education, support, and technical assistance in matters relating to bioelectromagnetics. See also the "Guide to Sources and Availability" on page 167.

Chapter 21

High-Tech H$_2$O: Supercharge Your Supplements

Your body is more than two-thirds water. Experts tell you to drink at least eight glasses of water a day to keep well hydrated — and with good reason.

Water carries almost everything you consume — the constituents of every herb, vitamin, food, or pharmaceutical — to the cells that need them. Every energy-boosting compound in ginseng, every immune-enhancing molecule in lactoferrin, every cancer-fighting phytochemical in broccoli, and every brain-enhancing, heart-protective, water-soluble nutrient in salmon... makes its way to your hungry cells via water.

In order to survive, renew, repair, and thrive, each cell in your body needs to consume, digest, and dispose of nutrients efficiently. Water carries nutrients into your cells and carries waste and toxins out.

It's no wonder, then, that for the past 30 years there's been an intense focus on the science of altering water molecules to improve their metabolic function. One scientist in particular, Dr. John Willard, discovered that changing the molecular structure of ordinary water resulted in a new form of activated water that was better absorbed — and thus enhanced the absorbability of nutrients consumed along with it.

He dubbed the resulting catalyst water "Willard Water." The ability of Willard Water to help the body assimilate nutrients and break down waste materials is supported by three decades of anecdotal evidence. Thousands have found that drinking Willard Water, or other catalyst waters, improves energy and overall health. In addition, many enjoy relief from symptoms and conditions ranging from high blood pressure to digestive and respiratory problems.

If you're interested in adding it to your health regimen, we have information on a new water catalyst, Crystal Catalyst, distributed by Higher Ideals Inc., a Utah corporation.

Crystal Catalyst, which is a concentrated solution of distilled water, sodium metasilicate, sulfinated castor oil, calcium chloride, and magnesium sulfate, is the only water catalyst with a United States patent, and the only one proven to shrink water molecules. This is critical, as the amount of nutrients your cells take in, as well as the amount of waste they let out, is limited by the permeability of the cell membrane, which only lets in or out a certain size molecule.

Imagine trying to walk through a narrow door with buckets of food. Obviously, you can only pass through with just so much at once. Water molecules attempting to enter a cell containing necessary nutrients are similarly restricted by the cell membrane.

Crystal Catalyst restructures the electrons of a normal water molecule, resulting in a new, smaller molecule. The catalyst creates a strong charge on the

nucleus of the atom to allow it to draw the other sub-
atomic particles closer together. This makes the water
molecule more compact and enables it to carry more
nutrients into your cell.

Catalyst water brings nutrients into the cell—nutrients the cell may not otherwise get. As a result, Crystal Catalyst is reported to. . .

- **improve the effectiveness of supplements.** In fact, Crystal Catalyst was developed primarily to increase absorption of
  tablets and capsules.
- **allow for greater and more efficient dis-
  posal of waste and toxins.** This is essential
  self-defense for today's toxic environment.
- **help your body's digestive process,** especially if you have problems with digestion
  due to depleted digestive-enzyme stores.
  Crystal Catalyst improves the absorption
  and transportation of minerals and
  microminerals that fuel enzymes. Thus,
  catalyst water may activate the enzymes
  you need to digest and process food.
- **reverse skin disorders,** such as eczema,
  psoriasis, as well as those related to allergies.
- **relieve arthritis pain.** Catalyst water has
  been used for thirty years as a treatment
  for arthritis. There are two possible expla-
  nations for this well-documented benefit:
  (1) Catalyst water reverses nutritional
  deficiencies, often the primary cause of
  arthritis. (2) Arthritis is often caused or

aggravated by acidic foods. Catalyst water has a pH of 12, which is extremely alkaline.

The term pH (percentage of hydrogen) is used to describe the acidity or alkalinity of a liquid or solution. Measured on a scale from 0 to 14, a pH of zero is extremely acidic, while a pH of 14 is extremely alkaline.

Many bacteria cannot live in a high-pH environment. Studies show that mixing catalyst water with disinfectants like Lysol improves their ability to kill bacteria. Catalyst water also enhances the effectiveness of antibiotics.

Crystal Catalyst also benefits the following:

- **Pets:** Animals who drink catalyst water may eat up to 50 percent less because they're absorbing nutrients better.
- **Laundry:** The smaller water molecules penetrate fibers better, allowing you to use less detergent.
- **Plants:** Cut plants, which are no longer able to absorb nutrients naturally (through their roots), can live an extra three to seven days when placed in a vase of catalyzed water.
- **Skin quality:** Crystal Catalyst rehydrates dry skin and improves the effectiveness of skin-care products.
- **The healing process:** It speeds the healing process of major burns, insect bites, sunburn, and rashes.

The manufacturer recommends using 1 ounce of Crystal Catalyst per gallon of pure distilled water to increase absorption of vitamins, minerals, herbs, and other supplements. For more information on Crystal Catalyst see the "Guide to Sources and Availability" on page 167.

A word of caution: Catalyst water may enhance the action of your medication, so space your medication and catalyst water two hours apart. Since Crystal Catalyst may increase the elimination of body toxins, you could experience a mild case of loose bowels, increased urination, or slight headaches. This is a temporary condition, lasting two to four days, and indicates that your body's natural cleansing process is working.

Chapter 22

Freeze-Frame: 60 Seconds to a Longer Life

As you know, the very first symptom of heart disease can be death. In the face of this grim reality, we're thrilled to be able to share with you an exciting new development in cardiology research. The Institute of HeartMath, a nonprofit educational and research corporation, has developed an assessment tool that helps doctors identify candidates for sudden cardiac death. Its research has also led to a technique that you can use. Not only can it help reverse existing hypertension, but it may also lower the chance of sudden cardiac death. It can also facilitate healing from coronary artery disease, angina, arrhythmia, and other cardiovascular disorders.

HeartMath has assembled an international team of superstars in the fields of cardiology, neurology, immunology, quantum physics, and psychology. These scientists have pioneered new biomedical research showing the direct relationship between mental/emotional balance and the healthy functioning of your heart, hormonal system, and immune system. They've unraveled the mystery of "entrainment," a natural phenomenon that occurs when two or more rhythmic systems, such as heartbeats and brain waves, synchronize.

Using the power of entrainment, HeartMath has developed a tool so powerful that the U.S. military is having its personnel trained in it. Heads of corporations are footing the bill for their employees, and alternative-health practitioners are flocking to Heart Math's training center in Boulder Creek, California.

This five-step process, called Freeze-Frame™, creates entrainment within your nervous system, producing proven results unlike those of any other self-relaxation method. At first, HeartMath taught the technique only in special seminars conducted at the institute in Boulder Creek. But it became clear that Freeze-Frame was extraordinarily effective, not only in lowering blood pressure but also in managing depression and anxiety, improving immune response, and providing other health benefits. So HeartMath produced a special videotape version of the method, which you can use in your own home.

When you first learn how to do Freeze-Frame, you might wonder how something so simple could possibly work, but don't be fooled. This is powerful stuff. One Fortune 100 company sent its employees—executives, administrative personnel, engineers, and factory workers alike—to learn this simple, straightforward technique. At the start of the study, 26 percent of the executive group had high blood pressure. Six months later, they all had normal readings. Even more astonishing, many reported the disappearance of long-standing symptoms like insomnia, headaches, indigestion, heartburn, and rapid heartbeat.

With Freeze-Frame, you "remove yourself" from your disruptive feelings, relax, focus, and entrain your heart rhythms, respiration, and blood pressure, all in five simple steps. Think of great athletes or dancers who are able to create a special, relaxed state of mental and physical focus in order to achieve a much higher level of performance. Now you can employ that exact principle with any mental or emotional activity. And the benefit to your heart is phenomenal.

Outsmart your body's primitive "fight or flight" responses

Using this new HeartMath technology, you can gain control of your autonomic nervous system — right down to the hormones you produce and the beat of your heart. With Freeze-Frame, you learn to induce entrainment, in which your entire system — heart, glands, organs, nervous system — works at maximum efficiency. It's no coincidence that moments of entrainment are associated with a deep sense of peace, fulfillment, and joy.

The results of HeartMath's research, published in the *American Journal of Cardiology*, the *Journal of Alternative Therapies*, and *Stress Medicine*, demonstrate conclusively that Freeze-Frame can lower high blood pressure and may reduce your risk of sudden cardiac death. And there are many more reported benefits, including increased energy and mental clarity, improved immune response, and relief from the symptoms of chronic fatigue and certain autoimmune diseases.

Some day, perhaps all hypertension—and many other diseases—will be healed with powerful heart-mind-body techniques like Freeze-Frame, instead of dangerous drugs and surgery. This is a medicine of the future—available today.

In addition to the Freeze-Frame program, Planetary Publications offers HeartMath books, audiocassettes, videotapes, and other educational materials, as well as original musical recordings scientifically demonstrated to improve hormonal, emotional, and immune-system balance. For more information, see page 167 for the "Guide to Sources and Availability."

Chapter 23

The Farabloc Blanket: Banish Pain Without Drugs

Despite 26 years of testing, double-blind studies, joyful testimonials, and solid professional recommendations, this exciting product remains mysteriously unknown.

It even works on the most excruciating kinds of pain: crushed bones, spinal column diseases, and even phantom limb pain—the very condition for which the fabric was invented.

The Farabloc blanket was developed in Bavaria by Frieder Kempe, a young inventor with a background in engineering and physics. Kempe was working to find a solution to the excruciating pain suffered by his father, an amputee.

Noting that his father's pain was worse on humid or rainy (low-pressure-system) days, Kempe theorized that positive atmospheric ions in the air were irritating the cut nerve endings in his father's stump. He reasoned that this external magnetic field was causing the nerve ends to send false signals to the brain—signals suggesting that the limb, along with the pain, was still there.

Over 50 different treatments had been tested on sufferers of phantom pain, and not one had worked well enough to be called a success: not surgery, drugs, ultrasound, hypnotherapy, psychotherapy, biofeedback — nothing.

After four years of research and development, Kempe tested the first prototype of the Farabloc blanket on his father. When the new invention eased his father's phantom pain, it was clear that Kempe's work had resulted in a revolution in pain relief.

After his initial success, Kempe set out to create a thinner, softer, more comfortable, more durable fabric. He tested cotton and linen versions but found them both less durable than the fabric he'd originally chosen: nylon. The final version, available today, is made of microthin threads of stainless steel wire woven with nylon. With proper care, this lightweight fabric, that looks and feels like linen, can last years.

Farabloc has been reported to relieve:

- joint pain
- rheumatic pain
- children's growing pains
- menstrual cramps
- sports injuries
- back ache
- postsurgical pain
- pain caused by cancer
- migraines and other types of headache

Kempe named the fabric Farabloc after Michael Faraday, the 19th-century French scientist who discovered electromagnetic induction, which later led to the invention of electricity. (The farad, an electromagnetic unit, was named in his honor.)

After five more years of testing, Kempe applied for and received a U.S. patent for his fabric. He then offered samples to amputees in Bavaria. They claimed it gave them "remarkable relief" from their pain. Soon after, Kempe immigrated to Canada, where he established the Farabloc Development Corporation.

Today, thousands of amputees all over the world — including Kempe's father, still living in Bavaria — are enjoying relief. The fabric has since been scientifically proven effective.

Skeptical scientists "couldn't believe the data"

In 1989, the British Columbia Health Ministry funded a two-year double-blind crossover study (Conine, et al., 1993) at the University of British Columbia. The study was run by Tali Conine, DHSc, PT, a professor of physical therapy at the University of British Columbia's School of Rehabilitation Medicine, and Dr. Cecil Hershler, a medical doctor and electrical engineer specializing in physical and rehabilitation medicine. A significant 61 percent of the first group and 62 percent of the second group reported the greatest pain relief when using Farabloc.

"We were so skeptical," says Conine, "we couldn't believe the data. We were at a loss to explain it in terms that scientists today understand. It was the most difficult article I have written in my life."

In the past five years, many professional health

Farabloc brings relief to thousands

Phantom pain

"When my son's pains started, I wrapped him, waist down, in the blanket, and the relief was immediate. The pains stopped and he relaxed. He has had no medication since I started using the blanket, and I have not used the T.E.N.S. machine once since."
— P.W. Squamish, B.C.

Migraine

"As a result of an old neck injury, I have suffered from terrible migraine headaches for many years. Nothing seemed to help until now, and the consumption of stronger and stronger painkillers affected my stomach in a very bad way.

"No more painkillers for me! At the slightest sign of an oncoming attack, I put the Farabloc on my neck and within a few minutes, the problem is gone. Even better, the intervals between the attacks used to last two or three days, while now I can go for longer and longer periods of time without any sign of it, almost like the problem is healing itself!"
—S.F., Coquitlam, B.C.

Sports injury

"On August 6, 1993, while playing tennis, I suffered a complete rupture of the Achilles tendon in my right leg. I had surgery, and my leg was then placed in a cast from the knee down. Very soon afterward, I began wrapping the Farabloc blanket around the cast during the day and at night. When I had the cast removed, the healing process was advanced much beyond the expectations of the orthopedic surgeon. In fact, I was able to walk without crutches within a couple of days of having the cast removed, and I had enough strength to walk on my tiptoes."

—A.S., Port Moody, B. C.

Chronic Shoulder Pain

"After an industrial accident in 1975, I was on workers' compensation and undergoing physiotherapy treatments every single day. I also received eight cortisone shots to reduce the constant pain in my right shoulder. The doctors told me at the time that there was nothing more they could do or provide for my pain in my right shoulder and that I would have to learn to live with it. Years passed, and the pain, always present, became so bad in 1989 that I could not sleep at night anymore. During the day, a daily work routine like shifting gears on my truck was almost unbearable. At that point, I was more than ready to try anything to ease the pain, but everything I tried failed to relieve my ache. After you recommended Farabloc, I asked myself 'What can I lose?' I used it as you recommended and just one week later my pain has eased off and my sleeping pattern therefore became normal again. Many thanks to you and your invention!"

—K. S., Burnaby, B.C

Migraine and menstrual cramps

"I have been using the Farabloc blanket for several months now, and I find it particularly helpful for my frequent migraine headaches. By wrapping the Farabloc around my neck, I get relief within a very few minutes. I also use it to relieve my menstrual cramps — it has helped me immensely."

—T. H., Langley, B.C.

Arthritis of the spine

"My husband, who has arthritis of the spine, is totally delighted with Farabloc and since using it has been able to sleep without discomfort in his back. He also finds that the relief now extends throughout the day even though he does not wear it at this time."

—A. P., Port Coquitlam, B.C.

organizations have begun regularly purchasing the Farabloc products — notably, the Insurance Corporation of British Columbia, the Ministry of Social Services, the Workers Compensation Board of Downsview, Ontario, and Veterans Affairs, Canada.

More independent studies are under way to determine how well Farabloc works for arthritis, delayed onset muscle soreness, and tendonitis, as well as sports- related injuries that cause swelling, especially in the knees and arms. Meanwhile, Dr. Gerhard Bach, a noted rheumatologist in the United States and Germany, has already established the use of Farabloc in other areas of pain relief.

The percentages listed below represent those who reported relief that was "good" or "very good":

- 81.3 percent: **phantom pain**
- 85.0 percent: **arthroses** (described as "painful disruptions of the functions of joints")
- 86.7 percent: **spinal column syndrome** (described as "static-degenerative changes to the spinal column ")
- 79.4 percent: other syndromes (shoulderarm syndrome, soft-part rheumatism, posttraumatic complaints, and complaints related to neoplasia)
- 63.6 percent: **chronic polyarthritis** (an inflammatory-rheumatic disorder characterized by chronic pain, swelling, and a reduction in the function of several small or large joints and tendon sheathes)
- 58.3 percent: **menstrual complaints**

How it works

The truth is Farabloc's painkilling action is still somewhat of a mystery. But there are a few working theories. As Kempe originally postulated, the blanket works to shield nerve endings from the aggravating effect of external electrical and magnetic fields.

Dr. Hershler, one of the doctors who led the first double-blind study on amputees, has also hypothesized that chronic pain is caused by alterations in blood flow deep within the muscles. He believes

Farabloc may actually increase circulation, thereby causing pain relief.

But there is another theory—that a slightly more mysterious healing mechanism is at work.

The truth about pain

Flowing from every swollen, torn, or inflamed tissue in your body are energy currents that send your brain the message to "feel pain." The best way to stop pain is to make those energy currents pass right out of you before they make it to your brain.

Since the late 1700s, scientists have been aware that our bodies generate electricity. Today, thanks to modern technology, we can evaluate health states by measuring various electrical waves. In fact, measurements of electrical output can determine just how healthy you are.

For example, studying electrical impulses in your brain helps to discern whether or not your brain is functioning normally. The EEG (electroencephalograph) test is used to uncover this information. When brain tumors are present, variations from the normal brain waves announce their presence. The same is true of heart and muscle areas. Scientists can even determine your sleep quality simply by measuring your "output" of delta waves, which are recorded in people who are enjoying a good, deep sleep.

Disperse pain currents with this "space age" pain reliever

As an electrically conductive fabric, Farabloc induces an electromagnetic field around the body (or around the limb for a local wrap). With the Farabloc fabric, the electrical "pain" energy generated within your body passes out of the body into the electromagnetic field of the blanket like an electrical ground or sink, thereby dissipating the energy that would otherwise travel up the sensory nerves as "pain."

What *doesn't* Farabloc work on?

Farabloc has not been shown to relieve pain caused by bruising, abrasion, or chronic fatigue.

What are the risks?

In a word, none. There is no risk to your health whatsoever, and there are no side effects.

Says Dr. Hershler, "I can be 100 percent sure that wrapping a Farabloc blanket around your limb does you no harm."

How to use it

To sustain pain relief, it is recommended that you begin using the fabric at the onset of pain. Wrap the garment, in two or three layers, around the painful area. Farabloc works best when placed directly on the skin and worn for a few hours from the time pain begins. In addition to wearing the Farabloc fabric as a blanket, you can sew it into socks, gloves, or sleeves, for example. You can even wash and air dry this thin, fine gray cloth (being careful not to wring it, to avoid damaging the fabric).

The fabric comes in four different sizes, which range from $70 for a handkerchief size, to $260 for a small blanket. See page 167 for the "Guide to Sources and Availability."

Chapter 24

Breast-Cancer Detection: Making Breast Self-Exams Easier to Perform

Vast amounts of time, energy, and print have been devoted to establishing the age at which a woman should begin regular mammogram screening. Meanwhile, many experts agree that the real question isn't when or how often you should have one but whether you should have one at all. In other words, is mammography — at any age — worth the expense and risk?

False positives are just one of the risks

Routine mammograms done on women in their 40s are estimated to produce false positive results in over a third of the tests. That means that out of 10,000 women tested, 3,000 to 4,000 of them would have a mammogram falsely interpreted as "suspicious." And most of those women would have to undergo further testing to determine if their breasts were, in fact, normal. False positives result in anxiety, unnecessary biopsy procedures, scarring, and distortions of the breast, further straining the future accuracy of testing.

Even worse, spokespeople for the National Institutes of Health (NIH) admit that mammograms miss 25 percent of malignant tumors in women in their 40s (and 10 percent in older women). In fact, one Australian study found that more than half of the breast cancers in younger women are not detectable by mammograms.

These false negative results, which can lull women into a false sense of security, are equally as dangerous as false positives. In a study from Sweden in which women younger than 55 showed a 29 percent higher death rate from breast cancer, researchers said, "Although this could be a random phenomenon, negative results of a screening mammogram may have falsely reassured some patients and led to a deleterious delay in diagnosis."

And even if mammograms are accurately interpreted, consider this: *The New York Times* quotes Donald Berry, a Duke University statistician, as saying that "98.5 percent of women in their 40s will get no benefit" from mammograms. "The other 1.5 percent will have their lives extended by 200 days."

A deadly distraction . . .

Monica Miller, a government relations specialist for alternative medicine, sees the whole debate about mammography as a deadly distraction from the abysmal state of breast-cancer care in the United States. Commenting on her personal choice to forgo mammogram screening, she says, "The idea of introducing radiation to radiation-sensitive tissue is absurd. If women start getting regular mammograms at 40, more cancers will be found because more cancers will be *caused* by the mammograms themselves."

A lot of sound and fury about one of the most questionable procedures in the fight against breast cancer

The worst thing about the mammogram debate is the possibility that, in the resulting confusion, women will be more likely than ever to do absolutely nothing to protect themselves. Attention has been diverted from the one procedure that allows women to take an active role in their own health care and that all experts agree is the key to the early detection of breast cancer: breast self-examinations (BSEs).

As one doctor puts it, "Women who do regular self-examinations can and do develop greater sensitivity toward their breasts and what is normal or abnormal than their doctors. In fact, between 50 and 60 percent of breast cancers are discovered by women themselves, either accidentally or through purposeful BSE."

There is an inexpensive and absolutely safe device that makes BSE much easier to perform and could increase its effectiveness. Unfortunately — and incomprehensibly — the FDA has refused to allow consumers direct access to this potentially lifesaving invention.

A maverick inventor's 11-year battle with the FDA

Earl Wright, an inventor from Decatur, Illinois, holds more than 150 U.S. and foreign patents. A former member of the U.S. Patent and Trademark Advisory

Committee, he was named an Inventor of the Year f-inalist in 1989 for his development of the Sensor Pad in 1984.

The Sensor Pad is a simple, inexpensive device — a latex-like pad 9.5 inches in diameter filled with about 2 tablespoons of medical-grade liquid silicone that allows the two layers of the pad to slip smoothly over each other. When held over the breast during a BSE, it makes the fingertips more sensitive by reducing friction and magnifying sensation.

- The Sensor Pad makes it easier for women to learn proper BSE technique and, by reducing friction, makes it easier to detect changes in breast tissue.
- It gives women confidence in their own ability to perform these important monthly exams and acts as a visible reminder to do them regularly.
- For many older women who are uncomfortable touching their own bodies, the Sensor Pad provides an "indirect" way to examine themselves.

However, despite evidence from women who claim the Sensor Pad saved their lives, despite the professional testimony of doctors and other breast-cancer specialists who agree on the need for this product, despite countless studies commissioned by the manufacturer showing it to be safe and effective, the FDA kept the Sensor Pad off the market in the United States for 11 years, citing a lack of scientific proof that the device works.

The Evolution of an Idea

In 1984, inventor Earl Wright was idly playing around with a half-deflated water balloon his grandson had left on the table. Rolling it back and forth over some grains of salt, it occurred to him that he could feel the salt right through the balloon — in fact, he could feel it better through the balloon!

Not yet sure of the possible applications of his discovery, Wright experimented with more than 80 combinations of different materials to find the one that enhanced his sense of touch the most. Then, he tried to figure out who might be helped by his new invention.

His first thought was to use it as an aid for reading Braille. People who are born blind learn this skill with relatively little difficulty. However, people who are newly blind often find it difficult to develop the fingertip sensitivity required for sightless reading. Earl went ahead with his plan to use his invention to help newly blind children and adults sensitize their fingers. And it worked. Still, he continued to search for other, broader uses.

When he realized its potential as an aid for breast self-examinations, the Sensor Pad was born. He reasoned that if the pad could increase the likelihood that a woman would correctly and regularly perform BSE, the odds of detecting and successfully treating early breast cancer would improve.

FDA classification keeps the Sensor Pad off the market

The FDA chose to classify the Sensor Pad as a "Class III medical device," a category that has included such invasive, high-tech inventions as pacemakers and heart-valve replacements — a category of products that, understandably, require extensive testing before FDA approval is given.

A Class III classification for the Sensor Pad? FDA spokesperson Sharon Snider defends this decision by insisting that the Sensor Pad poses an indirect threat. If it "fails to do what it's supposed to do," she says, "it could have very serious consequences for a woman: It could cost her her life."

However, no one is claiming that the Sensor Pad is anything more than a lubricating aid. Nancy G. Brinker, founder of the Susan G. Komen Breast Cancer Foundation, says, "There is no way you could convince me that doing a breast exam with a Sensor Pad could be any more harmful than not doing one at all — which is what happens with most women." She adds, "I think it's absolutely ridiculous that something that could be so potentially helpful to women is being kept off the market by government bureaucracy."

Finally, a victory — of sorts

The Wrights didn't back down. They truly believed in their product, and so they continued to fight, spending millions of dollars in the effort to get FDA approval. Then, just as they were about to give up, the FDA came through. Kind of.

Yes, the Sensor Pad is finally available. But you need a prescription to get one. And you can't get a prescription from your doctor and buy the pad at your local drugstore. Your doctor or local breast-screening center has to order it for you directly and give you in-person instructions on how to use it. Apparently, the FDA doubts the ability of women to follow written instructions.

Is this consumer protection?
Or a bureaucratic boondoggle?

In 1985, Earl and his son Grant were ready to market the Sensor Pad. They applied for authorization in Canada and got it within 30 days. They also got approval in Japan, Singapore, Korea, Thailand, and most West European countries. But when they asked the FDA for approval, they hit a roadblock.

The FDA kept asking for more and more information and more and more studies. "Ridiculous," says Grant Wright. "The Sensor Pad works on the same principle as soap and water — it reduces friction. Women are told to do breast exams using soap and water all the time. But you don't see the FDA asking for studies on that."

Still, the Wrights attempted to comply with request after request by the FDA. They were especially frustrated because they didn't consider the Sensor Pad to be a medical device and therefore doubted that the FDA had any jurisdiction over it.

Actions:
- Works on the same principle as soap and water, making fingertips more sensitive by reducing friction and magnifying sensation

Benefits:
- Makes it easier for women to learn proper BSE technique
- Makes it easier to detect changes in breast tissue

In 1988, after years of waiting, the Wrights consulted an attorney and were advised to start selling the pads directly to hospitals. The pads were enthusiastically accepted by both the medical community and their patients. In little more than a year, the Wrights' company, Inventive Products, sold more than 200,000 pads. Then, in 1991, the FDA got wind of this "unauthorized" activity and raided the company's headquarters, confiscated 30,000 pads, and, after a two-year legal battle, managed to bury the Sensor Pad even deeper in red tape.

Using the Sensor Pad

Your doctor or local breast-screening center has to order the Sensor Pad for you directly and give you in-person instructions on how to use it.

Chapter 25

Space-Age Water Filtration: Clean, Healthy Water — Finally!

Home water filters are designed to protect against contaminants that are unseen and mostly untasted. The damage done by these contaminants (lead, benzene, and chlorine, for example) can be catastrophic, but it may take decades or longer to become evident.

How water is purified

Water can by purified in three ways: through reverse osmosis, distillation, or carbon filtration. All of these methods have inherent weaknesses.

(1) Reverse osmosis: Reverse osmosis forces water through a membrane with pores so small that only water molecules get through. This process can even be used to turn salt water into freshwater, but not without the expenditure of large amounts of energy. Reverse osmosis is also slow, usually requiring a holding tank to store the accumulating clean water so that it can be used in quantity when needed.

The main problem with reverse osmosis is that everything is removed — including every beneficial trace mineral. Absolutely pure water (H_2O) may be "safe," but "safe" and "healthful" are not always the same thing.

In fact, there is a large body of research implicating "soft" water as a risk factor for cardiovascular mortality — while drinking water that is "hard" is consistently linked with lower mortality from heart disease. (Hardness is determined by the amount of calcium, magnesium, calcium carbonate, and other minerals dissolved in the water. Pure distilled water is extremely soft.)

(2) Distillation: Distillation is the oldest water purification process, and it removes all the good minerals as well as the contaminants. It's energy hungry, because the water has to be boiled, although an industrial-scale distillation plant can recover most of this heat energy. Even if pure H_2O were desirable, distillation would be the most expensive and least practical option for the domestic consumer.

(3) Carbon filtration: That leaves carbon filtration, the purification method generally favored for countertop use. Granulated activated carbon (GAC) is the material of choice for filtering out most organic contaminants. It has the necessary chemical (or "atomic") properties and, when properly processed, has a vast amount of surface area. One gram of GAC typically has about 1,000 square meters of surface area (about as much as 10 football fields). That explains why carbon-based filters can keep working for a long time before they begin to lose effectiveness.

But filtration with GAC is more complicated than

simply providing lots of carbon surface. It's also important to match the chemical structure of the carbon to the structure of the substance being filtered out. In other words, you can target particular contaminants by the specific type of GAC used in the filter.

So, obviously, the best filters for domestic use are designed to pull in the substances most likely to be problematic in domestic water supplies: chlorine, chloroform, and other chlorine derivatives; benzene and other hydrocarbons; and other volatile organic chemicals (VOCs).

The special problem of heavy metals

Metals like lead and mercury have been appearing in domestic water supplies, and their long-term effects can be deadly. They don't lend themselves to filtration by GAC, so any filtration system that stops with a carbon filter is leaving out an important part of the job.

But these metals can be removed by specially designed agents, such as certain types of ceramic material. In tests performed to satisfy the rigorous requirements for California certification, one type of countertop filter is proving to be extremely effective at removing lead, mercury, and other dangerous metals.

A space-age filter to the rescue

This filtration system was developed incorporating the same technology that NASA uses to purify

Choosing a Water Filter:
You Have to Be Scientific

When evaluating a water filter, you have to think qualitatively and quantitatively — there's no way around it. Nearly all filter manufacturers provide test results, but it's up to you to interpret them correctly. For example, the performance data provided by the manufacturer are based on a specific flow rate (that is, how many gallons per minute the filter processes). But keep in mind that filters become significantly less effective at higher flow rates. This means that if the test results are based on a very slow flow rate, or if you have high water pressure (which increases the flow rate), the test data will not accurately predict the performance of the filter in your home.

To get the best performance from your filter, be sure that the flow rate does not exceed the one used in the manufacturer's tests. To do this, place a bucket under your faucet, with the filter attached, and turn the cold water on full blast for exactly one minute. The amount of water in your bucket should be equal to or less than the gallon-per-minute rate specified in the literature. If your flow rate is too fast, you can slow it down by turning the tap only halfway on.

Find out what volume of water the system can clean before the filter needs to be replaced, but remember that the dirtier the water, the faster it will use up the filter. A very rough average is 1 gallon per day per person for countertop use. Better filter designs make it increasingly difficult for water to flow through the unit at the end of the filter's useful life, signaling that it's time to change your filter. Also, you'll want to consider the replacement cost of the filters.

If possible, compare the contaminants removed in the test report with those contaminants found in your own water supply. Many municipalities and state agencies can test your water for a nominal fee and give you an analysis. Check your local government listing. You can also send a sample for analysis after installing your filter, to be sure that it is performing adequately.

Finally, please note that countertop filters are only meant to filter cold water. Heat increases solubility and makes the water filter less effective. To filter hot water, you will need to install a "whole house" filter system, which filters the water before it enters your hot-water heater. In this case, your typical consumption rate will be 50-75 gallons per day per person. However, other potential hazards, such as chlorine gas released from hot water during showers, will be eliminated.

drinking water for our astronauts in space. It has now been specifically designed for household use.

The system, which uses the "Aquaspace" filtration compound manufactured by Western Water International, represents a huge advance in household water-purification systems. This material is approximately 70 percent granulated activated carbon and 30 percent aluminum-silicate ceramic. Don't be put off by the presence of aluminum. It's extremely inert in this form and does not end up in the water that passes through it. Elemental aluminum is the form that's to be avoided, and test results actually show a 96 percent reduction in aluminum in water filtered by the Aquaspace compound.

Actions:
- A water filter composed of a combination of 70 percent granulated activated carbon and 30 percent aluminum-silicate ceramic, it removes heavy metals (like lead and mercury) as well as most organic contaminants generally found in domestic water supplies.

Benefits:
- Unlike reverse osmosis and distillation, carbon filtration removes toxic materials from the water but leaves behind the beneficial trace.

The unique properties of this particular filter result in the removal of a fairly wide spectrum of dangerous metals. However, the lighter minerals associated with healthful spring water are allowed to remain. The

Aquaspace filter is also very effective in removing VOCs and chlorine, along with a number of other common contaminants. See the "Guide to Sources and Availablility" on page 167 for ordering information.

Guide to Sources and Availability

Due to their breakthrough, underground nature, many of the remedies presented in *Underground Cures* may not be readily available in health-food stores or other retail outlets. As a service to our readers, we have identified several high-quality, reliable sources for the products discussed in this book.

If you are interested in continuing to have access to the latest, most powerful discoveries and modern, underground treatments like the ones in this book, please turn to page 179 to find out how you can receive monthly *Members Alerts* from the Health Sciences Institute.

Anti-Homocysteine Products (Chapter 13)
Advanced Nutritional Products
1300 Piccard Drive, Suite 204
Rockville, MD 20850
Tel: 888-436-7200 or 301-987-9000
Fax: 301-963-3886

Healthier YOU
PO Box 9515
Lake Worth, FL 33466-9515
Tel: 800-350-7430 or 561-434-5525
Fax: 561-439-5173

Calcium Elenolate (olive-leaf extract) **(Chapter 4)**
Smartbasics
1626 Union Street
San Francisco, CA 94123
Tel: 415-749-3990
Fax: 415-351-1348

Catalyst Water (Chapter 21)
Higher Ideals, Inc.
2300 N. Main Street
North Logan, UT 84341
Tel: 435-752-1777 or 800-636-8644
Fax: 435-750-6738

Collagen Hydrolysate (Chapter 11)
Swansons Health Products
PO Box 2803
Fargo, ND 58108
Tel: 800-437-4148
Fax: 800-726-7691

DHA (Omega-3 fish oil) **(Chapter 15)**
Healthier YOU
PO Box 9515
Lake Worth, FL 33466-9515
Tel: 800-350-7430 or 561-434-5525
Fax: 561-439-5173

Emu Oil (Chapter 8)
Canyon Global Corporation
Canyon Ranch
Vanderpool, TX 78885
Tel: 830-966-3429 or 800-887-9499
Fax: 830-966-3399

Farabloc (Chapter 23)

Farabloc Development Corporation
3030 Lincoln Avenue, #211
Coquidam, BC, Canada V3B 6B4
Tel: 604-941-8201
Fax: 604-941-8065

Freeze-Frame (Chapter 22)

Planetary Publications
PO Box 66, Dept. FFVB
Boulder Creek, CA 95006
Tel: 408-338-2161 or 800-356-5325
Fax: 408-338-9861

Garum Armoricum (Chapter 5)

Smartbasics
1626 Union Street
San Francisco, CA 94123
Tel: 415-749-3990 or 800-878-6520
Fax: 415-351-1348

Infopeptides (Chapter 2)

The Right Solution
500 E. Cheyenne Avenue
North Las Vegas, NV 89030
Tel: 702-399-4328
Fax: 702-642-4491

Kava Kava (Chapter 19)

Lifestar Millennium, Inc.
2175 E. Francisco Blvd., #A-2
San Rafael, CA 94901
Tel: 415-457-1400 or 800-858-7477
Fax: 415-457-8887

Vitalmax Vitamins
710 E. Hillsboro Blvd., Suite 100
Deerfield Beach, FL 33441
Tel: 800-349-6977 (for information)
    800-815-5151 or 954-970-2022 (for ordering)
Fax: 800-866-4875 (for ordering)

Lactoferrin (Chapter 1)

Advanced Nutritional Products
1300 Piccard Drive, Suite 204
Rockville, MD 20850
Tel: 888-436-7200 or 301-987-9000
Fax: 301-963-3886

Smartbasics
1626 Union Street
San Francisco, CA 94123
Tel: 415-749-3990
Fax: 415-351-1348

Larreastat (Chapter 12)

Herbal Technologies
1674 Mountain Pass Circle
Vista, CA 92083
Tel: 760-598-2593
Fax: 760-598-5517

Liquid Oxygen Products(Chapter 14)

Healthier YOU
PO Box 9515
Lake Worth, FL 33466-9515
Tel: 800-350-7430 or 561-434-5525
Fax: 561-439-5173

The Right Solution
500 E. Cheyenne Avenue
North Las Vegas, NV 89030
Tel: 702-399-4328
Fax: 702-642-4491

Magnetic Field Therapy Devices (Chapter 20)

Bioflex, Inc.
3370 NE 5th Avenue
Oakland Park, FL 33334
Tel: 954-565-8500
Fax: 954-568-6117

Healthier YOU
PO Box 9515
Lake Worth, FL 33466-9515
Tel: 800-350-7430 or 561-434-5525
Fax: 561-439-5173

Medicinal Mushrooms (Chapter 3)
To find a distributor near you, contact:
Gourmet Mushrooms
PO Box 180
Sebastopol, CA 95473
Tel: 707-823-1743
Fax: 707-823-1507

Natural Progesterone Cream (Chapter 9)

Healthier YOU
PO Box 9515
Lake Worth, FL 33466-9515
Tel: 800-350-7430 or 561-434-5525
Fax: 561-439-5173

Natural EFX
100 N. Central Expressway, #350
Richardson, TX 75080
Tel: 972-644-7500
 Fax: 972-680-2311

Noni (Chapter 7)

The Right Solution
500 E. Cheyenne Avenue
North Las Vegas, NV 89030
Tel: 702-399-4328
Fax: 702-642-4491

Organic Germanium (Chapter 6)

Vitamin Connection
72 Main Street
Burlington, VT 05401
Tel: 802-862-2590 or 800-760-3020
Fax: 802-862-2459

Plant-Based Nutrition System (Chapter 17)

Green Kamut Corporation
3397 19th Street
Long Beach, CA 90804
Tel: 562-498-1998 or 800-333-0751
Fax: 562-498-9529

Plantago Major (Smoking Deterrent) (Chapter 18)

Bio-Nutritional Products
41 Bergenline Avenue
Westwood, NJ 07675
Tel: 201-666-2300 or 800-431-2582
Fax: 201-666-2929

Probiotics (Chapter 10)

Lifestar Millennium, Inc.
2175 East Francisco Blvd., #A-2
San Rafael, CA 94901
Tel: 415-457-1400
Fax: 415-457-8887

Healthier YOU
PO Box 9515
Lake Worth, FL 33466-9515
Tel: 800-350-7430 or 561-434-5525
Fax: 561-439-5173

St. John's Wort Products (Chapter 16)

Healthier YOU
PO Box 9515
Lake Worth, FL 33466-9515
Tel: 800-350-7430 or 561-434-5525
Fax: 561-439-5173

Smartbasics
1626 Union Street
San Francisco, CA 94123
Tel: 415-749-3990
Fax: 415-351-1348

Vitalmax Vitamins
710 E. Hillsboro Blvd., Suite 100
Deerfield Beach, FL 33441
Tel: 800-349-6977 (for information)
    800-815-5151 or 954-970-2022 (for ordering)
Fax: 800-866-4875 (for ordering)

Water Filtration System (Chapter 25)

Western Water International, Inc.
7715 Penn Belt Drive
Forestville, MD 20747
Tel: 301-568-0200

Index

HEALTH SCIENCES INSTITUTE

This book has been based on the research of the **Health Sciences Institute**. Our monthly newsletter is designed to give you private access to hidden cures, powerful discoveries, breakthrough treatments, and advances in modern, underground medicine.

Whether they come from a laboratory in Malaysia, a clinic in South America, or a university in Germany, our goal is to bring the treatments that work, directly to the people who need them. We alert our members to exciting medical breakthroughs, show them exactly where to go to learn more, and help them understand how they and their families can benefit from these powerful discoveries.

Members of the **Health Sciences Institute** have the opportunity to take advantage of special reports, incentives, and products. Subscribe now by calling the member services hotline at (410) 223-2611. Or just fill out the form below and return to:

Health Sciences Institute
105 W. Monument Street
P.O. Box 17560
Baltimore, Maryland 21298

- -

Membership Form

☐ **YES!** I would like a one-year subscription to the **Health Sciences Institute** newsletter at the special introductory price of $39. (That's 12 confidential *Members Alerts!*)

_____
Name

_____
Address

_____
City

_____
State/ZIP

_____
Phone Number
(in case we have a question about your order)

☐ My check is enclosed for $ _____ made payable to the **Health Sciences Institute**. (MD residents add 5% sales tax)

☐ Please charge my:
   ☐ Visa ☐ MasterCard ☐ AMEX

Card no.

☐☐☐☐☐☐☐☐☐☐☐☐☐☐☐☐

Exp. Date _____

Signature _____

this harmful effect. See page 70.

• Japanese people have a very low incidence of **colon cancer.** See why on page 56.

• See page 58 for the amazing nutrients that **stopped tumors** in tests at Albert Einstein College of Medicine.

• Did you know that, contrary to popular belief, eating the right amount of butter, eggs, milk, cheese, and well-marbled beef can actually **lower harmful cholesterol levels**? See page 67.

• This little-known, little-eaten food is a powerful cancer fighter. The National Cancer Institute published the results of a study that determined this food contains an active anti-cancer element with the power to slow the development of mammary tumors. Documented healing and disease-fighting effects of this nutrient include **treatment of aging, digestive upsets, prostate disease, sore throats, acne, fatigue, sexual problems, allergies,** and a host of other problems. See page 156.

• This vegetable may have preventive and even curative powers over cancer and is considered the first line of defense against cancer. See page 191.

• According to the National Cancer Institute, adding just 200 micrograms daily of this natural substance found in our soil might prevent cancer. Experts now say that cancer rates across the board could be cut by as much as 70% if the general population took this small amount daily. Japanse women who do have just one-fifth the rate of **breast cancer** of American women who don't. Learn what natural food contains this important substance on page 252.

You will find the answers to all of this and much, much more in *How to Fight Cancer and Win*. At the turn of the century, cancer claimed the life of one person in thirty. Today cancer kills one in five.

"Your book and the work of Dr. Budwig is truly great! I know of a woman in my church who had a brain tumor and became blind. After taking Dr. Budwig's formula, her sight came back! I met her mother just the other day—she told me her daughter is now free of cancer! Thank you." Ruth K.

"How to Fight Cancer and Win is a milestone in publishing history. I have never read a more down-to-earth, practical resume of cancer prevention and treatment. It's one of the most important books ever written on cancer and degenerative disease." Edward Steichen, M.D.

"My Prostate Problems Are Gone... Bless You"

Just released: the all-new, revised edition of *Miraculous Breakthroughs for Prostate and Impotency Problems*. This thorough healing guide for every man over 35 is now available to men who are concerned about their prostate—and to women who are concerned about their men.

Surgical procedures on the prostate are among the most commonly performed operations in America. With impotence and incontinence as common side effects, it's no wonder men fear prostate disease and surgery. This book defeats fear by telling all sides of the story and gives every man reason for the hope of return to vigor and vitality. It also tells you what doctors often don't—for many men, nature offers far better alternatives than surgery.

• For example, one patient decided to take the natural healer and tonic revealed in Chapter 3 before scheduled prostate surgery. Very shortly after beginning the healing doses, the man noticed his prostate troubles were gone. His urologist canceled the surgery!

• In another case, one patient named Bill had a prostate so swollen that he visited the restroom every 20 minutes. Yet, in less than a month of the natural remedy on page 35, Bill's symptoms eased, and within two months, he was sleeping through the night again.

• Another patient, Larry R., was told his prostate should be surgically removed. He took two natural supplements revealed on page 36 and noticed improvement within 10 day. In a month, all signs of prostate problems had disappeared!

Even if your prostate is healthy, you should follow this natural way of male health as a preventative measure. The table on page 38 tells exactly what to take.

Father Hohmann, a priest, was diagnosed with terminal prostate cancer. His doctor considered his case hopeless and told the priest to make his peace and retire. But he wasn't ready to die. Using an herbalist's prescribed remedy given a page 59, Father Hohmann found a cure "nothing less [than a] miracle."

Have your prostate battles left you feeling hopeless? See page 60 for the most potent natural remedy of all, able to help even cases declared hopeless. This super-potent male remedy has helped bring relief to the toughest prostate complaints *without doctors, drugs, or surgery*! Not getting enough of the one essential mineral given on page 26 can lead to infertility, and, in severe cases, impotency.

Dr. Rudolf Sklenar, a German medical doctor, popularized the male potency elixir named on page 55 after he noticed the robust health of elderly Eastern European and Russian peasants. The men boasted of their lovemaking prowess well into their nineties.

"I'm not a health expert or any type of nutritional specialist; I am just an average guy—a guy who used to suffer from prostate disease. But thanks to William Fischer's latest book, I am no longer bothered by my prostate. I spent literally years searching for a doctor who could help me, but I found no relief. Finally, I gave up and resigned myself to living with the pain. My wife bought me a copy of *Miraculous Breakthroughs*, but I was sure it would be of no use. Boy, was I wrong!

"There is so much sound advice, I can't imagine any man not finding something that agrees with his body and his lifestyle. I was thrilled to discover that two products worked especially well for me. The answer to my problem was so simple." Mr. J.C.B., New York.

"Several years ago I developed some problems with my prostate gland. The troubles looked innocent enough at first, but they eventually grew and the situation got more seri-ous. Someone loaned me a copy of the original edition [of the book].

"Well, before I knew it, my problem had eased up. My doctor was surely surprised (shocked would be a better word), and I made sure I checked with him every so often. My prostate problems are gone. I'm happier than I've ever been and believe it or not, I feel I have the energy of someone half my age! Bless you!" Mr. C.H., California

The objective of the book is to help men prevent prostate problems and cancer. For those who are quietly suffering with these conditions, the goal is to find ways to relieve the pain, reverse the disease, and restore the body to <u>vibrant natural health</u>.

Miraculous Breakthroughs for Prostate and Impotency Problems is the owner's manual for the male body. You owe it to yourself and to your loved ones to read this book and discover the healing possibilities it offers.

Slow down aging with this Russian longevity formula

Fight cancer with this Italian wonder "drug" that has been featured in The New England Journal of Medicine

Eat fatty food (including red meat) and still lower your risk of heart disease using this proven German method

This Turkish salep will make your love life wild again

Natural Health Secrets from Around the World

More Than 1,600 Proven Remedies You Can Use at Home

As you read this, more than eight million people in Sweden are slashing their risk of heart disease by as much as 60%. Over one billion more in China and Japan are medically "bullet-proofing" their bodies against cancer. Countless others are getting rid of back pain, impotence, headaches, hair loss, and fatigue. And all without surgery or dangerous prescription medications. They are using the healing power of natural medicines and drugs that have been developed over thousands of years in countries all around the globe. For example:

• In India, **arthritis pain** is routinely eliminated with this "miracle" root. Add it to your diet and you too may begin to live pain-free…See page 113.

• This Chinese tea remedy really works for **menstrual cramps**. (And it's available in your local health food store.)…See page 364.

• People from Mexico, Saudi Arabia, Cambodia, and Burma use this versatile miracle treatment to cure **impotence, increase energy, boost stamina,** and **cure headaches**… See page 286.

Finally available in America

Until now information about alternative health remedies such as these was not publicized in America. And no wonder. The U.S. medical establishment is very uncomfortable with the fact that millions of people in all different parts of the world are living healthier, happier, and longer than most Americans—and without expensive and dangerous drugs and surgical procedures.

Dr. Glenn Geelhoed, an expert on international medicine, worked with a group of researchers to create a useful and practical guide that any American could use to take advantage of the preventive and curative traditions that other cultures have been using to keep themselves healthy for hundreds of years.

The result is the 650-page *Natural Health Secrets* volume, a book dedicated to the idea that there is so much you can do before your body fails—so much you can do to prevent disease and live longer—without high-tech, intrusive procedures. You can do so much today—right now—to rid your life of pain and recover the energy and vitality of your youth. And it's all within easy reach.

Safer and less expensive

The fact is, these natural healing methods are often safer and much less expensive than mass-market drugs. Time and again, natural remedies have proven effective where the conventional approaches have failed. And every one of these 1,600 remedies can be found or used at home. For example:

• Russians can drink all night and still **avoid hangovers**—their secret is surprisingly simple.

• Don't let **headaches** keep you from enjoying life…use the super-fast cure discovered by North Africans—it may be the best cure yet!

• Find out how Italians smoke, drink, and eat plenty of pasta…yet still have a lower incidence of **heart disease** than Americans.

• Check your kitchen cupboard—you might have this powerful American Indian aphrodisiac on hand to use whenever, however, and how often you wish.

• Look younger with this Caribbean cure for **wrinkles.**

• Relieve **back pain** with an exotic fruit ointment popular with pain sufferers in the Fiji islands.

• Boost your **energy level** without caffeine or drugs—ancient Olympians used this safe, high-energy stimulant to improve stamina and performance.

• In the depths of the Burmese jungle people routinely live past 100—their secret not only guarantees **longevity** but keeps them **virile, energetic,** and **healthy** year after year.

• Add this Seminole Indian remedy to your diet and you may never come down with a **cold** again.

• This Russian treatment for **hemorrhoids** gives quick, long-lasting relief—yet it costs a fraction of the price of commercial preparations.

In recent years, the public has been clamoring for more information and access to natural cures from overseas. American medical institutions are now researching many of these natural methods and medicines. The results verify that many natural cures do have substantial scientific validity. For example:

• A report in *Annals of Internal Medicine* concludes that garlic, a Chinese doctor's staple, lowers **cholesterol**.

• Some scientists believe that bark from this 100-year-old European tree contains a chemical compound that might provide a cure for **cancer**.

• A Harvard Medical School team reported that an extract from this southern "weed" helps treat **alcoholism**.

• A **natural sex stimulant** used by men in West Africa for centuries has been tested for effectiveness by the Stanford Medical School—and the results are very encouraging!

Why is Natural Health Secrets so different?

To tell the truth, I don't believe there's another resource anywhere that reveals so many useful alternative natural remedies. Other health references—even those published by America's top health publishers—tend to focus on Western medicine and American approaches to health and healing. There's nothing wrong with this except that these offer a very limited perspective. There's a whole world of natural remedies and cures available to you. Why shouldn't you know about them?

I have no doubt that this book will show you secrets that could make your life—and the lives of people you love—healthier, happier, longer. *Natural Health Secrets* may very well be the most useful resource for natural medicine available today. And for a limited time, you can own your own copy for just $29.00.

Call Today! 1-800-851-7100 • Order Code: NHS-NHUCB

Or, send us this coupon along with your payment of $29 plus $5 shipping and handling for each book to the address below. Your copy of *Natural Health Secrets from Around the World* will be delivered to your door.

❏ Please send me _____ copies of *Natural Health Secrets from Around the World*.

Name _____

Address _____

City _____ State _____ Zip _____

Phone (____) _____
(In case we have a question about your order)

❏ I have enclosed my check or money order for $29.00 *plus* $5.00 shipping and handling for each copy, made payable to Agora Health Books. (MD residents add 5% sales tax.)

❏ Charge my: ❏ VISA ❏ MasterCard ❏ AMEX

Card No: _____ Exp. _____

Signature:_____

This book comes with a *100% Satisfaction Guarantee*. If you are not fully satisfied, you may return it within one year for a complete refund. No questions asked.

Agora Health Books • P.O. Box 977 • Frederick, MD 21705-9838

NHS-NHUCB